GOD'S DIET PLAN: Seek Him First

A 31-Day Devotional Guide for Healthy Eating and Weight Loss

Linda Ross Shoaf

ISBN-13: 978-1-7337052-0-2
ISBN-13: 978-1-7337052-1-9 (eBook)

The author is a licensed/registered dietitian nutritionist. Content of this book is not intended to replace professional medical advice. The author claims no responsibility to any person or entity for any liability, loss, or damage caused or alleged to be caused directly or indirectly as a result of the use, application, or interpretation of the information in this book.

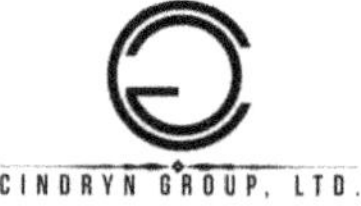

Cindryn Group, Ltd.
Horn Lake, MS

Library of Congress Control Number: 2019901889

Interior design by Rhonda Dragomir: www.dragomirgroup.com.
Cover design by Kristie Koontz: kristiekoontz.myportfolio.com.

Dedication

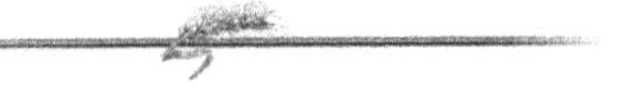

Dedicated to all who struggle with weight loss or healthy eating and desire to live a healthier lifestyle

Acknowledgements

My sincere thanks to Jeris Hamm for her
encouragement and assistance
in making this book possible.
Thank you to all members of the KCW
critique group, past and present,
who had any part in reviewing these words
and offering encouraging comments.
A special thanks and gratitude to my husband David
and our daughters Kathryn and Cynthia
for their continuing support and encouragement.

Table of Contents

Preface

Most likely, you are reading this devotional book because you have an interest in a healthier weight, or you desire to help someone close to you find the courage to shed excess pounds. Weight is a complex issue. One thing we do know, since the 1960s, the number of obese adults has more than doubled and continues to rise. Why is that? With the increased number of those experiencing excessive weight has come greater susceptibility to diseases and illnesses.

According to health care standards, a Body Mass Index (BMI) between 19 and 24 is the preferred weight for optimal health (See Body Mass Index Appendix 1). A BMI between 25-30 is considered overweight. Figures above 30 represent obesity (See Classifications of Obesity Appendix 2). To determine our starting point, the BMI tells us where we are and where we need to be for a healthy weight.

We often hear grim health statistics for obesity. Physicians may advise us to lose weight to help some physical problem. Many of us want to look better and believe losing a few pounds will accomplish our goal. There's nothing wrong with that either.

Sometimes we try over and over to lose weight and fail. We overeat or make unwise choices. And if honest, we know certain foods are tempting, yet we yield. Are we doomed to weigh more than health charts suggest is healthy? Some of us hit a plateau and nothing we do moves that scale downward. For a few of us, illness or medications hinder our efforts. A small number are predestined by heredity or genes to remain overweight—but a very few. While past studies insisted the obese can be just as healthy as their thin brothers and sisters, current research tells us that isn't so.

How does God feel about our weaknesses when we make unwise food choices? Will he punish us if we fail to lose weight? What about those who struggle and can't get pounds off? When we do our part, God understands.

First, know that God uniquely created each of us. He loves us and desires what is best for our lives, every part, including size. God wants us to stay as healthy as possible.

In these thirty-one days of devotionals, we will 1) come to a greater understanding of God's unending love, 2) explore how to care for our bodies, 3) learn God's plans for our lives through encouragement, 4) praise God for the insights and blessings we experience, and 5) find his will for us.

Each devotional begins with a Scripture focus. "Prayer with Purpose" follows each devotional text to guide our petitions and fellowship with God while "Thoughts to Ponder" leads us to reflect on our actions. "Lesson for Life" provides the key to move forward each day in a closer walk with God's desires for our lives.

Each devotional concludes with "Digging Deeper" which lists questions for meditation and application in our daily lives. These are designed for individual use or combined after each section for group study to draw deeper into God's Word and reflect on the spiritual aspects of the week's devotionals.

The back of the book includes nutrition information for further study. It provides useful facts to nourish and maintain our bodies for service to God.

Together, let's study the Scriptures to determine if God cares if we are fat. And then we can work and pray together for answers to become nourished in body and spirit.

Dear friend, I hope all is well with you and that you are as healthy in body as you are strong in spirit.
3 John 1:2

Part I
God's Love

1 Image of His Love

Then God said, "Let us make human beings in our image, to be like ourselves . . . ." So God created human beings in his own image. In the image of God he created them; male and female he created them.
Genesis 1:26-27

When we gaze into a mirror, it reflects our image and the many characteristics of our ancestors. We see a newborn and soon decide who the baby looks like. The turned-up nose brings images of its mom or the bushy eyebrows resemble dad's. As the child grows older, we recognize various traits of family members. From two people God gave this child many characteristics of generations past.

After God created this world and everything in it, he declared it good. God, the one and only architect, fashioned earth. In six days, he formed light and darkness, land and sea. He completed this marvelous planet and formed humans to share his universe which continues today as he uniquely molds each of us.

Not only did he make us, but he created us to be like him. Just as that tiny infant acquired traits of its parents, God molded us into his image with a soul and spirit. Genesis states, "Let us make human beings in our image." Us refers to the Trinity, the three in one; God, Jesus, and the Holy Spirit. John in his gospel says, "In the beginning the Word [Jesus] already existed. The Word was with God, and the Word was God. He existed in the beginning with God" (John 1:1-2). Jesus, as part of the Trinity, was God who made everything through this Word, and in turn, gave life to everything created.

Just as we as parents take pleasure in watching our children grow and develop their abilities and personalities, our Heavenly Father loves watching us become more like him. He made us, men and women, to rule over this earth, and his handiwork pleased him. We teach and influence our children's actions during formative years and desire for them to develop into healthy adults. In the same way, God cares about our every thought and action, even to what we eat. How could we ever doubt his unconditional love?

Prayer with Purpose:

Lord, thank you for creating me in your image. Keep me mindful that every life is a product of your almighty hand and reflects you. Amen.

Thoughts to Ponder:

- God created men and women after his own image.
- Regardless of the characteristics inherited from ancestors, we are formed in God's image.
- God's love for each of us is unconditional.

Lesson for Life:

Out of inexpressible love, God created mankind in his own image.

Digging Deeper

1. What do you see as the correlation between God's creation of the heavens and earth and his creating of mankind?

____
____
____
____
____

2. How does knowing you are formed in God's image affect your decisions and actions?

____
____
____
____
____

Perfection of His Love

I pray that your love will overflow more and more, and that you will keep on growing in knowledge and understanding. Philippians 1:9

God formed Adam, the first human, like himself for a heaven-earth communion. Adam was the perfect human symbolism of God, yet he needed a compatible companion. Eve became his female counterpart. God created them for fellowship with himself to share in a close, personal way. He placed his human creations in a perfect garden to daily walk and talk with him. Satan's lure through deception caused Adam and Eve to break God's command about eating fruit from the tree of knowledge of good and evil (Genesis 3:1-7).

The intimate relationship between God and mankind changed forever. Through disobedience, this perfect couple with their gift of free will introduced sin into a flawless world. Despite mistakes, God still loved them. But the sin of Adam and Eve did not go unpunished. Their sin passed forward to all future generations. Yet, God's love never ceased.

God as our potter fashions us as clay in his hands (Isaiah 64:8). He chooses unique characteristics and abilities for each of us and molds us into the best we can be. However, he allows us freedom to make choices. Just as Adam and Eve chose sin over an unblemished world, so we have the independence to make life-changing decisions. While God desires for us to make healthy food choices, we choose what we eat, often with consequences. Jesus said in the book of Matthew that we were to be perfect as our Father in heaven is perfect (Matthew 5:48). Because of sin, that is impossible. But God loves us even in our imperfections. He is willing to direct and provide every good thing, including decisions about food (See Strategies for Developing a Better Eating Pattern Appendix 3). Almighty God desires to commune with us through prayer and the study of his Word.

Prayer with Purpose:

Lord, my creator, you have fashioned me like yourself for fellowship. Keep me from sins that may interfere with a godly relationship with you. Amen.

Thoughts to Ponder:

- God expects obedience from his human creations.
- Sin disrupts our fellowship with God.
- Actions affecting our bodies reflect either praise or disregard for how God made us.

Lesson for Life:

Disobedience to God in every aspect of life may result in unpleasant consequences.

Digging Deeper

1. When God created man and woman, they were perfect. Food was the instrument used to tempt them and cause the downfall of mankind. How do you visualize and describe Eve's relationship with God before and after her sin?

____
____
____
____
____

2. Why would Eve believe Satan instead of God?

____
____
____
____
____

3. In what ways do you demonstrate disobedience to God through your lifestyle, and what steps are you willing to take to become more obedient?

____
____
____
____
____

3 *Wonder of His Love*

I will praise thee; for I am fearfully and wonderfully made: marvelous are thy works; and that my soul knoweth right well.
Psalm 139:14 KJV

There she lay—our newborn—cradled in my arms quietly sleeping. Earlier, her wails indicated a healthy set of lungs as she made her debut into this world. My husband and I examined her tiny, slender fingers and the wisps of thin blond hair that framed her face. She was ours. I nurtured her for nine months as this beautiful body formed inside me. We began this journey with God as creator of our perfectly healthy little girl. And she was hungry. Two tasty fingers on her left hand became her solace while awaiting food and other comfort. We felt unbelievable joy and love for our child.

Like most parents, we taught and encouraged our daughter during her formative years. She grew independent to choose her own activities and food. In the same way we wanted the best for our child, God wants us to grow physically, emotionally, and spiritually. He wants to cradle us in his loving arms and care for us.

The Lord said to Jeremiah, "I knew you before I formed you in your mother's womb. Before you were born, I set you apart"

(Jeremiah 1:5). He continued by telling Jeremiah that he had set him apart as a prophet. Likewise, we are set aside for his purpose.

God wove together the inmost parts of our bodies with stunning workmanship. The complexities of our form demonstrate his unending love. He knows our hearts and thoughts.

The psalmist invited God to search his heart and examine him and to point out anything that might offend the Spirit (Psalm139:23-24). We have every cause to praise God for the way he formed us. Whatever we do, wherever we go, God's Spirit follows his creations, from the heavens to the grave. He is there to guide and support us. Can we present ourselves before God and ask, as did David, for the Lord to examine us and point out every offence to the Spirit?

Prayer with Purpose:

Lord, thank you for making me the way you have. I may lack the physical attraction or mental abilities of others, but you made me as perfect in your sight. Help me nurture within myself what you have created. Amen.

Thoughts to Ponder:

- Everyone is made perfect in God's sight.
- Whatever our physical features or mental capacity, God cherishes us and wants us to tend to the bodies and minds he gave us.
- God desires for us to show appreciation for our perfections and perceived imperfections.

Lesson for Life:

Every person's life is precious in God's sight.

Digging Deeper

1. God knows you completely. He formed you as his perfect creation. Nothing is hidden from him. In what ways can you show appreciation of how God made you?

   ____
   ____
   ____
   ____

2. What role does food have in your relationship with God, our Father?

   ____
   ____
   ____
   ____

3. When you perceive certain foods as harmful to your body, how does that affect what you eat?

   ____
   ____
   ____
   ____

4. Why do you think God does or doesn't care when you choose foods that may prove harmful?

   ____
   ____
   ____
   ____

4

Proof of His Love

For God so loved the world, that he gave his only begotten Son, that whosoever believeth in him shall not perish, but have everlasting life.
John 3:16 KJV

Growing up I had a favorite aunt. Her closeness to my mother, her big sis sixteen years her senior, made her special to me. She looked up to my mother, and they kept in close contact. Perhaps one cause for my warm bond with her resulted because she often reminded me of her presence when I was born. As with most situations, the more time we spend with those we love, the stronger the relationship grows. God was with us from the time we were created. He wants to remain with us and for us to remain with him.

While we may like some people in our lives better than others, God doesn't have favorites. He doesn't treat individuals from any ethnic group differently. He doesn't show partiality between men and women or show favor based on incomes. And he doesn't distinguish between those who are short, tall, skinny, or fat. He loves each of us beyond measure, and the Apostle John tells us how God proved his love.

John, known as the beloved disciple, seemed to have a special relationship with Jesus. But Jesus did not love him any more than the other eleven. As the youngest disciple, he had the advantage of seeing what others wrote in their gospels and chose to record the life of Jesus from a very different perspective. Who was this Jesus he described?

John begins his gospel—the good news—referring to Jesus as the Word. Through his existence, Jesus brought light—or eternal life—to everyone. But that's not all John told us about this Word—Jesus. Why would he leave heaven and come as an infant to live among mortal humans? God allowed his Son to come to earth and sacrifice himself so we could have the opportunity to live forever with God. What greater proof could we have of his love?

You may have known and believed that for a long time. If you struggle or worry about how you look or how much you weigh, remind yourself of God's everlasting love. If you haven't known about that adoration, now is the time to accept God's son and live in the joy of knowing how much you are loved.

True fellowship with God comes only through belief in Jesus' sacrifice for us. It surpasses any human bond that could ever exist. What else can possibly matter?

Prayer with Purpose:

Dear God, thank you for proving your love and making a way for me to live with you forever. Amen.

Thoughts to Ponder:

- God loves us all the same, regardless of our size or shape.
- God allowed Jesus to come to this earth to give us the opportunity to live with him in fellowship forever.
- Jesus willingly accepted the task of living among mankind even though it cost him his earthly life.

- If God loved us that much, we have no cause to doubt we are worthy of such love.
- The greatest present we can ever accept is God's gift of eternal life.

Lesson for Life:

No greater love exists than God's sacrificial love for mankind.

Digging Deeper

1. God loved you so much he sacrificed his own son for your sins so you could have eternal life. How are you willing to prove your love for him?

____

____

____

____

____

2. What role, if any, does forfeiting unhealthy food play in your worship of God?

____

____

____

____

____

5 Strength of His Love

I pray that from his glorious, unlimited resources he will empower you with inner strength through his Spirit. Then Christ will make his home in your hearts as you trust in him. Your roots will grow down into God's love and keep you strong.
Ephesians 3:16-17

As a teenager I grew up around cotton fields where a plant we called "shoestring vine" (trumpet vine) plagued our efforts to salvage cotton stalks from its tendrils. Although a menace to those who picked cotton by hand, the domesticated plant produced lovely trumpet-like flowers and beautiful seed pods for fall arrangements. Even a plant unwanted by farmers had a useful purpose to others. This plant had long, sturdy roots that grew deep into the soil.

We may become entangled in poor lifestyles that affect health and well-being. Problems and issues often distract our thoughts and actions. Like those cotton stems entwined with that pesky weed, little things may play havoc with our judgment and undermine trust in our loving God. We yield to different temptations—even poor food choices (See Foods to Limit Appendix 4). Sometimes drastic circumstances may change our lives forever.

Like the trumpet vine, God wants to wrap us in tendrils of his love, not to harm but to protect us from worldly evil. Through our trust in him, we develop strong root systems that grow deep into God's love to keep us from the wiles of Satan's forces. He empowers us with inner strength to withstand temptation's snares. The more we sense his devotion, the more we worship him. The deeper the love in our hearts for him, the more we live in Jesus.

Whether in major disasters of life or in small everyday irritants, God helps us grow stronger in his love to withstand earthly trials and make wiser decisions.

Prayer with Purpose:

Lord, I pray that through your glorious unlimited resources my love for you will grow deeper each day as I depend on you for strength. Amen.

Thoughts to Ponder:

- God can replace worldly difficulties that entangle our lives with his tender arms of love.
- Trusting in God helps us overcome everyday temptations, even the unhealthy foods we often eat.
- The deeper our roots grow into God's love, the more we will put our trust in him.

Lesson for Life:

God's love empowers us with inner strength to keep us strong.

Digging Deeper

1. Our spiritual strength comes through God's love for us and our love for him. In what ways does the Holy Spirit empower you in making life's choices and efforts to eat healthy foods?

____

____

____

____

____

2. How will you apply your love for God, especially as it relates to what you eat?

____

____

____

____

____

Depth of His Love

And may you have the power to understand, as all God's people should, how wide, how long, how high, and how deep his love is.
Ephesians 3:18

God created an amazing Earth. Most of it we may never see. Our planet extends to unbelievable depths and rises above the clouds. The Mariana Trench of the Pacific Ocean with a depth of more than 35,000 feet is the deepest part of the ocean. Can we imagine? Eight of the ten highest mountains are found in the country of Nepal. Mount Everest, a part of the Himalayan Mountain Range, is the tallest mountain at more than 29,000 feet high.

The Nile River in Africa is the longest river in the world, followed by the Amazon in South America and the Yangtze in Asia, each about 4,000 miles long. But the Amazon takes first prize for width, spanning nearly seven miles during the dry season and almost twenty-five miles during the wet season.

As amazing as these wonders are, they cannot compare with God's love. The Apostle Paul prayed that the Ephesians would have the power to understand the width, length, height, and depth of God's love. When we understand that, we will come to the reality of how much he is willing to do for us.

Each new day, God's love remains constant. If he loves us that much, what keeps us from loving the bodies he gave us? If our physical form has become less healthy due to our neglect or abuse, do we love him enough to change how we care for his creation? Regardless of how busy or distracted we are in our many activities, let's remind ourselves that he is always there. He will guide us, even in the food we select to eat (See Healthy Eating Patterns Appendix 5).

Prayer with Purpose:

Creator of all, empower me with understanding of your great love. Help me to experience its depth in my daily life. Amen.

Thoughts to Ponder:

- Just as the creation of our world is difficult to comprehend, so is the depth of God's love.
- When we seek guidance to improve life choices, God willingly helps.
- We can express daily appreciation and devotion for God even through what we choose and have to eat.

Lesson for Life:

Because God's love is immeasurable, so also should be our commitment to him.

Digging Deeper

1. The Apostle Paul prayed that the Ephesians would have the power to understand God's love. How do you get that power?

____

____

____

____

____

2. In what ways does God's affection for you or your adoration for him relate to what you eat or drink?

____

____

____

____

____

3. How does understanding God's love help you choose a better lifestyle, including the foods you eat?

____

____

____

____

____

7
Power of His Love

May you experience the love of Christ, though it is too great to understand fully. Then you will be made complete with all the fullness of life and power that comes from God.
Ephesians 3:19

With the advent of electricity, life became easier as we relied on electrical power for machines to do much of our physical labor. I recall my mother whipping egg whites by hand for her melt-in-your-mouth angel food cakes. How much easier for me to dump those egg whites into a bowl and let my heavy-duty mixer whirl away.

And what about dads who chopped down huge oak trees with an ax instead of powerful chain saws? Electrical current surges through our homes to power appliances, lights, and many electrical gadgets.

In the same way, the Holy Spirit empowers us with inner strength. The Spirit within us is greater than the spirit who dominates this world (1John 4:4). It surges through us to deter Satan and "self" from causing poor or immature judgments. This advocate helps us, even with simple daily tasks and decisions.

The Gospel of John tells us that without God, we can do nothing (John 15:5). This verse can apply to numerous areas of life. Many of us need prompting to eat as we should. The Holy Spirit within us strengthens our resistance to food temptations that fail to provide our bodies with needed nourishment. We can turn to the Holy Spirit for the power to conquer poor eating habits (See Food Exchange List Appendix 6).

Prayer with Purpose:

Lord, help me experience your love and be made complete with the fullness of life. May the Holy Spirit empower me to know and choose healthy diets. Amen.

Thoughts to Ponder:

- When we experience Christ's love, he makes us complete with the fullness of life.
- Making right choices about foods we eat begins with knowledge.
- God, through the power of the Holy Spirit, leads us to trustworthy information about foods and nutrition.

Lesson for Life:

When we ask, the Holy Spirit directs us to appropriate nutrition information and gives us power to improve eating habits.

Digging Deeper

1. The power of the Holy Spirit within you conquers more than you can ever do alone. That force far exceeds the capability of Satan. In what way does accepting the Holy Spirit's power and revelation help you to avoid dangerous eating patterns?

   ____
   ____
   ____
   ____
   ____

2. How will you allow the Holy Spirit to assist in planning a better daily eating strategy?

   ____
   ____
   ____
   ____
   ____

Part II
God's Temple

8 Identify the Temple

For we are the temple of the living God.
As God said: "I will live in them and
walk among them. I will be their God,
and they will be my people."
2 Corinthians 6:16

Suppose God gave us a building no one else could use and said, "This is a structure made especially for you. It will be yours for several decades. This edifice is special to me so make every effort to keep it in good repair and use it in a way that will please me." How would we treat that building knowing it was a gift from God, and he expected us to be a good steward of his possession? Would we carelessly throw junk into that structure? Would we allow it to become damaged or destroyed because of our actions or inactions? If we thought that what we did to our bodies affected God's Holy temple, would we change a few things? Maybe a lot of things?

Our bodies *are* God's temple. He knows every cell in our bodies and hair on our heads, and he desires for us to value this human structure. He cares how we treat temples.

A teacher attempting to make a point gave the following illustration: "If you went to the doctor and he told you to lose weight or you would die within six months, you would do it."

I appreciated the point she tried to make, but her conclusion was inaccurate. We hear warnings almost daily from health professionals, friends, or media about how we are killing ourselves by the foods we eat.

How can we ignore the effects of unhealthy diets? Poor eating habits have been linked to diabetes, many types of cancer, and an increased possibility of heart disease, which often leads to earlier death. Next to smoking, obesity is the greatest environmental factor—those things we often choose to do to ourselves—leading to earlier death (See Effects of Obesity on Health Appendix 7).

Everyone will die sometime of something, but we are caregivers for this one and only temple God gave each of us to house our spirits. When we identify our bodies as God's handiwork, perhaps we will appreciate and take better care of ourselves.

Prayer with Purpose:

Dear God, this body you gave me is your holy temple. Thank you for this form made especially by you. Help me to treasure your gift and identify my body as yours—because it is. Amen.

Thoughts to Ponder:

- God, in the form of the Holy Spirit, dwells within each of us.
- What we put into our bodies indicates how we feel about God's temple.
- The care we give our bodies shows whether we think of them as worthy or unworthy vessels.

Lesson for Life:

When we recognize our bodies as God's temples, we understand why they require optimal care.

Digging Deeper

1. God developed your earthly body as his holy temple. What does the phrase in 2 Corinthians 6:16 "For we are temples of the living God" mean to you?

   ____
   ____
   ____
   ____

2. Identify ways you often harm your body. If overeating is one of the negative points, list five ways you can change that habit. Post your list in a prominent place, such as your refrigerator door, as a reminder.

   ____
   ____
   ____
   ____

3. Consider how the foods you eat affect your body. Reflect on or discuss how the way you treat your body may reflect how you feel about God. What changes will you make to more readily glorify the temple God gave you?

   ____
   ____
   ____
   ____

9 Nourish the Temple

I am the one who answers your prayers and cares for you. I am like a tree that is always green; all your fruit comes from me.
Hosea 14:8

We lived several states away from my husband's home place. When his mother died, I never knew what happened to the household belongings. His unmarried sister lived a short distance from their mother and took care of her personal effects.

Years later, we bought a second house between his hometown and mine where we could stay while visiting relatives in the area. We needed furniture. I vaguely recalled an old bedframe in his childhood home that would be perfect for a guest room. I asked my husband, "What happened to the contents moved from the homestead decades ago?" I was horrified to learn the furniture had been stored in a grain bin, surrounded and almost obscured by weeds, in the middle of a field. With his sister's permission, we retrieved salvageable pieces and had them repaired and refinished. What should have been valued items would never be the same due to years of unintended neglect.

Yogi Berra said, "If you don't know where you are going, you'll end up someplace else." When it comes to health, where do we want to end up? If we don't know, we may end up physically someplace we don't want to be. God doesn't want us to allow our earthly form to deteriorate like the family pieces of furniture. Neglect of our bodies could keep us from the health we could have had. However, even when we have postponed appropriate care, there's hope. Vitality may improve when we make positive changes. We may delay physical conditions from getting worse. God can and will "be health to [our bodies] and strength to [our] bones" (Proverbs 3:8 NKJV).

Prayer with Purpose:

Lord, my spirit lives and the Holy Spirit dwells in this holy temple you gave me. Help me to honor you by the care I give my body. May I choose foods that nourish so I remain as healthy as possible. Amen.

Thoughts to Ponder:

- Neglect of our bodies often results in deterioration of health.
- A continued lifestyle of poor choices may damage our bodies beyond repair.
- God is always available to help with decisions, even those about foods we eat.

Lesson for Life:

How well we care for God's temple often results in the quality of life we live.

Digging Deeper

1. Attention to your body impacts quality of life and may contribute to how long you live. On a scale of one to ten, how would you score the care you give your body?

   ____

2. State at least five ways you could improve your score.

   ____
   ____
   ____
   ____
   ____

3. What positive changes will you make in eating habits to improve or maintain your physical well-being?

   ____
   ____
   ____
   ____
   ____

4. How would you interpret Hosea's word that God is like a tree and all our fruit comes from him? How does this verse apply when you neglect proper care of God's temple?

   ____
   ____
   ____
   ____
   ____

10

Dwell in God's Tent

For we know that when this earthly tent we live in is taken down (that is, when we die and leave this earthly body), we will have a house in heaven, an eternal body made for us by God himself and not by human hands.
2 Corinthians 5:1-4

In his first letter to the Corinthians, the Apostle Paul identified their bodies as God's temples. He urged them to show reverence toward this housing of the soul and spirit. Because God made and formed our bodies, they deserve utmost attention.

In his second letter to them, he referred to their bodies as tents—our short-lived lodging on earth. Much like the familiar tents common to the people of Paul's day, they recognized them as temporary accommodations. Paul wanted them to understand that in eternity, God will transform their earthly tents into eternal dwellings. He continued to explain that current bodily tents don't compare to future heavenly vessels planned for them and for us.

Human forms grow weary and wear out. We may long for a more functional and up-to-date one in the same way we desire to cast aside old garments and put on new clothing (2 Corinthians

5:2). But Paul assured the Corinthians that after we leave this earth, we will have new bodies. While we remain on earth, God expects us to tend to the ones we have.

Our heavenly bodies will never decay or need physical sustenance as mortal tents do. How do we care for these earthly vessels? Earth-bound bodies sustain many trials and abuse, often at our own hands, including poor diets that fail to nourish. For most of us, abundant food supplies abound. Modern medicine and conquered deadly diseases have extended lifespans. Yet, we often punish our worldly tents with unsuitable foods. Until we get to heaven, the wise among us will choose nutritious fares to maintain our health. Healthy foods in the right proportions usually increase quality of life and longevity.

Whether we think of our bodies as temples or tents, they house who we are—God's remarkable creations. The size, shape, or color of the body God gave us doesn't supplant our significance or responsibility to treat and care for whatever he has given to glorify him.

Prayer with Purpose:

Lord, whether my soul and spirit are sheltered in a temple or tent, it was created by you for your purpose. Help me to eat the healthiest foods and initiate the best health practices. Amen.

Thoughts to Ponder:

- God provides an earthly and heavenly dwelling to house our souls and spirits.
- Our bodies need the right nutrients and care to sustain our life while on earth.
- The foods we eat influence how long we dwell in our earthly bodies.

- Staying healthy depends on knowing and consuming the best sources of nutrients.

Lesson for Life:

How we care for our bodies can reveal our dedication to God.

Digging Deeper

1. Paul compares the bodies of the Corinthians to earthly tents which God will exchange for heavenly dwellings. Define earthly tents compared to eternal bodies.

____

____

____

____

2. How can you develop healthier eating habits while you remain on earth?

____

____

____

____

____

3. However you perceive the type vessel God gives—temple or tent—how important do you consider the food you eat?

____

____

____

____

____

4. Health problems often exist regardless of how we eat. Assess those physical problems that plague you and list ways foods may help your condition improve either directly or indirectly.

____

____

____

____

____

11

Protect the Temple

You will keep him in perfect peace, whose mind is stayed on you, because he trusts in you.
Isaiah 26:3

While we owned the old house near my home area, I would often steal away to visit relatives or work on writing tasks. I felt safe in that old place—except when thunderstorms occurred. Gusts of wind rattled the windows. Branches of large trees bumped and shook the house. I doubted the electrical wiring was trustworthy. Whenever lightening flashed nearby, the fuse box hissed and popped causing me to double check for fire.

Late one evening, a thunder cloud rolled in unexpectedly. A sudden streak of lightening and clap of thunder startled me. I quickly checked outlets, appliances, and every possible place to assess damage. There was none. Once again, I felt safe and secure—but not my body. Mentally I was fine, but I could not believe the effect the unexpected interruption had on my entire system. My whole body shook. My heart continued to pound rapidly, even while in my mind I felt quite safe.

My experience was short-lived, and eventually my body caught up with my mind. But what happens when we endure little tensions for weeks on end? We may think everything is fine, but those pressures take a toll on health. Mentally we feel everything is under control, but our bodies aren't convinced. Stress has a price.

Can we avoid stress? No. But we can learn better ways to face the anxieties of life. The psalmist writes, "As pressure and stress bear down on me, I find joy in your commands" (Psalm 119:143). Do we have the same joy as the psalmist?

How do worries affect our health or how much we weigh? Stress-eating occurs when we attempt to fulfill emotional needs with food (See Guidelines to Control Emotional Eating Appendix 8). Stress impacts appetite and the amount we eat. Traumatic periods may increase desires for comfort foods—those special goodies or dishes which brought comfort in childhood.

Some foods have a calming effect. Foods high in fat and sugar temporarily make us feel better. Those who eat during stress—emotional eaters—tend to eat calming foods because they improve mood. In time, the chemical pathways in those diets link mood changes with eating high-fat, high-sugar foods. The association continues to grow stronger, increasing the amount of comfort foods needed to get the desired feelings. This cycle can result in excess weight. Eating foods to help our emotions becomes out-of-control and results in more stress instead of less.

Chronic stress causes the abdominal area to store more fat which is known to increase risks for diabetes, heart disease, and cancer. Stress may even counteract the effects of a healthful diet. Does God care? Of course, he cares. Finding measures to reduce anxieties helps protect our bodies—God's earthly temples (See Managing Chronic Stress Appendix 9).

Prayer with Purpose:

Lord, help me to identify stresses in my life—to list them one by one—and seek your guidance to approach each in the most appropriate way. Reveal those areas where I use food as an escape and help me to alter my eating habits. Amen.

Thoughts to Ponder:

- Stress can be a major factor in uncontrolled eating.
- Psychological and physiological aspects of stress may cause weight gain.
- Most areas of stress do not immediately go away, and many will never change.

Lesson for Life:

How we respond to the many stresses in life may reveal our relationship to God.

Digging Deeper

1. State or discuss specific ways God can help you grow spiritually during stressful times.

   ____
   ____
   ____
   ____

2. List positive steps you can take to reduce the stress level in your situation.

   ____
   ____
   ____
   ____
   ____

12

Defend the Temple

Be strong in the Lord and in his mighty power.
Put on all of God's armor so that you
will be able to stand firm against
all strategies of the devil.
Ephesians 6:10-11

It had been a hectic day. The holidays rapidly approached. In preparation, I made batches of two favorite party mixes. Usually I avoid even tasting them because I have trouble stopping after just a taste.

I succumbed to the temptation. Sure enough, one bite led to another, then another, and another. I gorged myself, even though I wasn't that hungry. Sound familiar? While I'm not a binge eater, I was on that occasion.

Like individuals under stress, binge eaters tend to eat foods high in sugar and/or fat. Leading temptations include pasta or bread. Other craving are sweets, fatty foods, or salty snacks. Many of us may think we fall into that category at times. Nearly half of women occasionally crave chocolate. Does that make us binge eaters? Like my one-time lapse, infrequent cravings don't necessarily result in a binge eater or a food addict.

When we plunge headfirst into food temptations, there's no need for despair. If it remains infrequent, hope reigns. However, some of us may drift beyond binge eating to become food addicts and cause harm to God's temple. For the most part, food addiction is self-diagnosed. No official definition exists. Why some people seem to become addicted to food is unclear. It could be environmental influences, learned behavior as a coping mechanism, or inherited traits.

Food addicts share many common characteristics with substance abusers and alcoholics. The brains of food-addicted obese people resemble those of drug addicts. They experience physical, mental, and emotional craving and a chemical addiction to food. Half of individuals with eating disorders also abuse alcohol or illicit drugs, complicating the problem (See Binge Eating and Food Addiction Appendix 10).

Is Satan the culprit? While causes may result from altered brain function, Satan can present situations to weaken resistance. Strength to avoid threatening circumstances related to food addiction comes from the Lord. The Holy Spirit within us is greater than evils in this world (1 John 4:4). We can seek appropriate help. God may lead us to professionals trained in food addiction problems. We can also ask for God's mercy to shield us, like a coat of armor, to resist the urges and temptations of food. Whatever we need to fight food addiction, God will help us prepare for battle. Trust him.

Prayer with Purpose:

Lord, help me to stand firm against Satan's strategies to food addiction. Grant me the armor to withstand misuse of food. Amen.

Thoughts to Ponder:

- Continual use of food as a crutch can result in serious eating problems.
- God's armor of truth, righteousness, peace, and faith is always available.
- Use of God's armor helps shield us from misuse of food.

Lesson for Life:

God wants to shield us against misuse of foods that may harm his temple.

Digging Deeper

1. What are specific ways the Holy Spirit can help you avoid Satan's snares related to what you eat?

____

____

____

____

____

13 Value Life

Teach me how to live, O LORD. Lead me along the right path. . . I am confident I will see the LORD's goodness while I am here in the land of the living.
Psalm 27:11, 13

George and Clarence in the movie *It's a Wonderful Life* paint a fantasy picture of what it would be like if we had never been born. George faced a crisis. He saw no way out. God sent Clarence, a not-so-successful angel, to help him recognize the value of his life and thereby earn his wings. Through the revelation of what the situation would be if he had never been born, George learned the significance of his existence. In the process of Clarence bringing this about, Clarence earned his wings.

Many of us occasionally feel like George. In my teen years, I remember dropping to the sofa and wishing I had never been born. I have no idea what in my young life prompted such thoughts. I had loving parents, and as the youngest, rarely wanted for anything.

But even as adults, we may have fleeting experiences like George. We bristle at snide comments about our appearance. We may sense rejection, whether founded or not, and endure cruel comments from others. Can we face one more day with excess weight and endure the tiredness that comes from dragging around extra pounds? We wonder if life is worth the effort.

What changes would there be had we never been born? Many of us find a Clarence who points out our significance. Even if we feel as though others don't care or understand us, God loves us unconditionally and wants whatever is in our best interest, including our diet.

Life is tough. Some mornings we want to turn over and close out the world. Problems and responsibilities may overwhelm us. When I face those days, I repeat numerous times, "This is the day the Lord has made; [I] will rejoice and be glad in it" (Psalm 118:24).

The psalmist petitioned God to teach him how to live. Have we asked God to teach us? The psalmist wanted his Maker to lead him along the right path and was confident of God's goodness. When we question the worthiness of our lives, are we seeking to see God's goodness? How can we question his call or fail to recognize his purpose for a full life whether we are age eight or eighty? As long as we have breath, we have value because we are his creation.

God desires for us to recognize the importance of each new morning and praise him for what he will accomplish every day through our lives. We are worthy in his sight. That's enough.

Prayer with Purpose:

Lord, help me to rejoice knowing you will sustain me throughout the day. Give me confidence in your goodness during the remaining days of my life. Amen.

Thoughts to Ponder:

- We serve an important purpose for God each day.
- Whatever problems we face, God knows and has a plan for the remainder of our lives.
- God makes each new day and wants us to enjoy it.

Lesson for Life:

We can celebrate each day assured that God knows our inner thoughts and will direct every aspect of our lives.

Digging Deeper

1. When attempting to lose weight, how do you overcome feelings that God has abandoned you?

   ____
   ____
   ____
   ____
   ____

2. How does weight affect your feelings about your daily life?

   ____
   ____
   ____
   ____
   ____

3. Reflect on people in your life like Clarence who have been important to you. Recall a time when you helped someone who was disenchanted and distraught about living.

____

____

____

____

____

4. When you feel despondent like George, what do you do to change your destructive inner attitude?

____

____

____

____

____

14

Honor Each Promise

But if you fail to keep your word, then you will have sinned against the LORD, and you may be sure that your sin will find you out.
Numbers 32:23

In my 20s, I was hospitalized briefly for tests. While awaiting my turn, healthcare workers talked among themselves about a patient across the hallway. She was scheduled for a glucose tolerance test to determine a diagnosis for diabetes. If positive, her physician would prescribe medications to help control the disease. That procedure requires avoiding any food after midnight prior to the test. Fasting blood is taken from patients, and then they drink a measured amount of glucose followed by blood draws at intervals to determine the glucose blood level at different times.

Somewhere along the process, nurses learned that my neighbor-patient, who was also a nurse, laughed about fooling all the medical staff. She had skipped the fasting part and ate a high-sugar breakfast. Of all people, she knew better. Her training told her blood sugar levels could not be accurate because of the added food, especially sugar. Why would she do that? I don't know what the medical personnel decided, but her ploy to eat despite instructions jeopardized results.

Why do we deliberately sabotage the very things that will keep us going? Most of us would not put regular fuel into our cars if the manual called for high octane premium gasoline. But we think nothing of putting less healthy foods into our bodies. Choices may keep us from feeling well, or they may eventually cause serious health problems.

The Book of Numbers gives an example of the perils two Israelite tribes faced if they failed to do what they promised and the rewards they would receive if they kept their word. They wanted to remain in Gilead across the Jordan River from the promised land of Canaan. At first, Moses was furious. The two tribes assured Moses they would help the other tribes conquer Canaan. Moses warned that if they failed to keep their word, their sins would be sure to find them out (Numbers 32:1-6, 16-27). These tribes kept their word, but what happens when we ignore promised consequences?

Often, we assure ourselves, families, or physicians we will lose weight. If we neglect to do so, health issues may result. When weight remains because of our broken commitment, we don't get by with failing to keep our word. God gave us one body, and there's no second chance for a new one. Wiser food selections may improve and renew tissues and cells to help us live a healthy and prolonged life. We may think we can get by without following dietary guidelines, but eventually our bodies let us know we have only fooled ourselves.

Prayer with Purpose:

Lord, forgive me when I deliberately treat my body in unhealthy ways. Help me not to sabotage my physical well-being through unwholesome eating and other harmful habits. Amen.

Thoughts to Ponder:

- As sure as our sins eventually become known, poor food selections may bring about unwanted physical conditions.
- God wants us to honor our bodies by eating healthy foods.
- Taking care of ourselves honors God while actions that deliberately harm our bodies disrespect him.

Lesson for Life:

Showing respect for our bodies demonstrates reverence toward God.

Digging Deeper

1. How would you respond if your child failed to keep a promise and committed actions that could be dangerous, even life-threatening?

____
____
____
____
____

2. What do you see as the correlation between keeping your word and honoring God by what you eat?

____
____
____
____
____

3. How often have you made New Year's resolutions to lose weight or eat healthier? What prevented you from keeping your word?

   ____
   ____
   ____
   ____
   ____

4. What steps will you take in the future to choose a better diet?

   ____
   ____
   ____
   ____
   ____

Part III
God's Encouragement

15 The Answer to Hopelessness

So encourage each other and build each other up, just as you are already doing.
1 Thessalonians 5:11

Decades ago my surgeon informed me that I had a breast lump and needed a surgical biopsy. Everything went well, and I was thankful the results were negative for cancer. As the doctor, who had a quiet sense of humor, discharged me he said, "If you are looking for sympathy, I can tell you where to find it."

"Where is that?"

"In the dictionary."

We both had a good laugh. But through the years, I have often thought about his words. My surgeon was right. Have we needed someone to share our burdens or concerns and felt as though the only place to find comfort or sympathy was in the dictionary? At times, we attempt to share our deep troubles with family or close friends only to find disappointment. They aren't interested. Or they make light of something important to us.

Maybe we were taught to hide our feelings. If so, we may hurt alone without seeking comfort from those who care about us. We all need someone.

Sometimes it isn't sympathy we seek or a need fulfilled but a small smattering of encouragement. In the Bible, the title Ecclesiastes means Teacher. The writer knew about hopelessness. This person, wise and successful throughout life, now felt all was pointless. He wrote that the sun rises and sets, then repeats itself, time and again. The wind blows in circles. The sea never gets full. How hopeless. Life has no purpose (Ecclesiastes 1:5-8). The writer continues with a litany of futilities—life, wisdom, pleasure, work, political power, and wealth. Despite a life of prosperity and success, those areas of importance no longer mattered.

What do lack of sympathy and a discouraged old man have to do with weight or eating right? As diet after diet fails us, we often feel hopeless and could appreciate sympathy and encouragement from others.

We are more likely to overeat when out with others. However, friends can be our greatest encouragers. The author of Ecclesiastes recognized the importance of companionship. He pointed out two are better than one and three are even better (Ecclesiastes 4:9-12). Isn't that true when we face difficulties or want to lose weight and nothing happens? Empathy from a couple of friends can be priceless. True friends support us when we share how desperately we need to lose pounds for health reasons. Likewise, we can encourage them to eat healthier selections to keep or improve their physical well-being.

Maybe an acquaintance in our group is waiting for us to speak out. Taking a stand empowers us. It's a type of self-encouragement. Once we take that courageous step, it emboldens us to move forward by eating foods we consider best for our health. At the same time, we become an inspiration for those who witness our commitment.

I traveled with a group of professional women to Florida for a national board meeting. At dinner, every one—except me—

ordered wine. Instead, I ordered my usual beverage of choice, hot tea. After the meal, one of the women I met at dinner confided in me that she had not wanted wine but ordered a glass when she thought everyone else planned to. Because I made a conscious choice to drink a different beverage, the following evening my new friend skipped the wine. The same can happen with other high-calorie foods. When we decline a food or beverage to avoid excess calories, others may follow.

It's hard when people tease or consider us different. But my experience has taught me that people appreciate and admire those who stand up for themselves in a polite way. The least we can do is try. Our boldness serves to encourage ourselves while we inspire others. Our confidence just may be the answer to hopelessness.

Prayer with Purpose:

Thank you Lord for those in my life who encourage me in my battle to consume fewer calories. Help me to reassure others in their efforts to eat healthier, even as I boost confidence in myself. Amen.

Thoughts to Ponder:

- Encouragers create healthy relationships.
- Encouragement negates feelings of futility.
- Self-encouragement can pay dividends to us and others.

Lesson for Life:

While encouragement is one of the gifts of the Holy Spirit, it is something all of us can practice.

Digging Deeper

1. What do you do when you fail to lose weight and despair sets in?

____
____
____
____
____

2. Based on this devotional "The Answer to Hopelessness," list positive steps you will take to counter hopelessness.

____
____
____
____
____

16

Seek God's Plan

You can make many plans, but the Lord's purpose will prevail. Proverbs 19:21

Our grown grandchildren live a distance from us. Occasionally, I send a text to keep in touch. Most of the time, I add a Scripture verse at the end.

One granddaughter, completing her nursing degree, shared with me her ambivalence about work and career. She planned to continue her education at some point, but she was undecided about which degree would be best for her, whether or not she should work a while first, and what God had planned for her future.

I sent a text concluding with the verse above. She immediately responded and thanked me for the encouragement. Of course, I want what is best for all my grandchildren. But I hope to encourage them by sharing what God already knows. His purpose will prevail.

We need encouragers in our lives, whether for a major event or for everyday concerns about our bodies. It's important to associate with folks who understand our dilemma and willingly encourage us by their words and deeds. If wise, we avoid people who choose to ignore our health needs or criticize and discourage our efforts.

How do we feel when eating with others who order tempting desserts even when they know our weaknesses and our desire to avoid high-calorie foods? What emotions surge when someone tells a "fat joke" or makes an off-handed comment about weight? Those people aren't helpful for physical or emotional well-being. Instead we can seek individuals who can and do empathize without preaching or scolding. Many times, others fail to stop and consider the impact of their words. Too often we allow negative remarks and actions to influence our plans for healthy eating.

Likewise, if prudent, we guard our tongues from disparaging judgments. I often wonder how many people I have encountered who needed a glimpse of God's plans through me—and I failed.

What plans do we initiate to acquire healthier habits and appropriate weight? Do we stay the course for healthy eating, or do we vacillate between sometimes and never? What is God's purpose for us concerning care of our bodies? "We can make our own plans, but the LORD gives the right answer" (Proverbs 16:1). We may realize the right answer for our lives is to take responsibility to stay within our eating plan with the Lord's help. When we "commit [our] actions to the LORD. . .[our] plans will succeed" (Proverbs 16:3).

Think how compliments from others elevate our spirits. Regardless of what we face, someone close to us or even a stranger who utters an encouraging word can change our day. Unfortunately, the same is true for discouraging words. Negative comments have an even greater effect than positive ones.

God rewards efforts to maintain optimal health. Will we seek his plans for our physical well-being and work with him? Or will we allow thoughtless people or Satan's temptations to thwart our attempts to reach a healthy weight?

Prayer with Purpose:

Lord, help me to rely on you with all my plans. May I become an encourager to others. Show me individuals to avoid who may frustrate my attempts at losing weight. Amen.

Thoughts to Ponder:

- God's plans for us are better than any we could make for ourselves.
- Encouragers bless us as we struggle at eating a healthier diet.
- Critical people destroy our confidence.

Lesson for Life:

How we feel about ourselves and our weight may hinge on the kinds of people with whom we associate and our willingness to follow God's perfect plan for us.

Digging Deeper

1. Reflect on ways you have sensed the Holy Spirit directing you toward specific plans for your life.

   ____
   ____
   ____
   ____
   ____

2. Share examples of individuals who have encouraged you in your plans, especially in areas of a healthier lifestyle.

   ____
   ____
   ____
   ____
   ____

17

The Power of Words

A word fitly spoken is like apples of gold in pictures of silver. Proverbs 25:11 KJV

I walked into the restaurant where former classmates gathered for a class reunion. The first person I encountered was a close friend in high school. We had not seen each other since the previous reunion, at least a decade earlier.

"You've gained weight," she said.

Taken aback, I mumbled something about my added girth.

She seemed to recognize her faux pas and responded off-handedly, "We have all changed."

In high-school I was the skinny kid who probably looked malnourished. Now decades later, the impact of slowed metabolism, health issues, and medications had taken its toll. Controlling my weight had become more difficult. Yes, I wanted to lose weight, but remained thankful for my health.

How do we respond to those who feel the need to point out our weight-gain even when it is a slip of the tongue? Or those who cheerfully tell us how much better we would look if we lost a few pounds? We know that! Reasons for too much weight vary. We usually know when it is a result of eating too much or choosing high-calorie foods. Even then, comments can be painful. But when weight results from issues that seem beyond our control, it hurts.

When I laughingly shared my reunion experience with my daughter who understood my plight, she didn't find it as funny as I did. She judged this person she had never met because of her lack of sensitivity. But like my friend who commented without thinking, likewise we humans often fault others for weight and similar issues.

While I sought to find humor in the situation, comments about weight aren't funny. We feel like responding as Job did to his less-than-helpful friends who accused and condemned him when he needed them the most. He said,

> "I have heard all this before." *Oh, haven't we.* "What miserable comforters you are! Won't you ever stop blowing hot air? What makes you keep on talking? I could say the same things if you were in my place. I could spout off criticism and shake my head at you. But if it were me, I would encourage you. I would try to take away your grief. Instead, I suffer if I defend myself, and I suffer no less if I refuse to speak" (Job 16:2-6).

Job's words echo how we may feel around certain family members or friends. Wouldn't we love to respond as Job? What if we criticized them in some way? Our words could be as hurtful to them as theirs are to us. Job's message is powerful. Do we encourage friends during their time of distress in attempts to lose weight?

At this point, Job became defensive instead of forgiving. I suspect we would, too. But for our own sake, it's best to set aside injured feelings, and like Job, encourage others in similar plights.

How do we defend our situation or dismiss unthinking friends or those boorish people who seem to delight in hurting others? Can or do we pray honestly and sincerely for them?

Through God's grace we can overcome thoughtless words, advice, and criticism. Thank God for those blessed words fitly spoken by caring people. They are powerful means of encouragement.

Prayer with Purpose:

Dear God, unkind words about my weight sometimes hurt. Restrain and replace my sin and guilt of unkind words with those as apples of gold. Amen.

Thoughts to Ponder:

- Words can be a powerful force of encouragement or discouragement.
- Thoughtless words harm us both emotionally and spiritually.

Lesson for Life:

When we can't change the circumstances, we can change our reactions.

Digging Deeper

1. Recall and share episodes of discouragement from family or friends and how you responded.

   ____

   ____

   ____

   ____

   ____

2. Reflect on positive ways you will react in the future.

   ____

   ____

   ____

   ____

   ____

18 Attitude to Encourage

And we are confident that he hears us whenever we ask for anything that pleases him. And since we know he hears us when we make our requests, we also know that he will give us what we ask for.
1 John 5:14-15

The well-known children's book, *The Little Engine that Could*, made its debut as part of a sermon in the early 20th century. Many revisions and rewrites occurred through the years, but the focal point remained. A determined little engine took on an impossible task and encouraged itself to successfully complete the challenge.

What was so heroic about the little locomotive? As the story goes, the pint-sized switch-yard engine sat in a small railyard. Every day he moved smaller cars and engines into different positions for extended jaunts across the countryside. When a larger engine could not be found to take a much-needed load of several cars across the mountain, the last resort was the tiny choo-choo. Out of desperation, the long train asked the little fellow if he was willing to attempt the task. He immediately took on the challenge and began the difficult assignment chanting "I think I can, I think I can."

If the authors had added backstory about the other trains, it could display negative reactions of the rail cars or other engines. How many would encourage him? Most would have predicted failure. But the small choo-choo mustered up courage and self-confidence. Slowly he neared the top of the mountain, straining and pulling. He chocked and gasped. For a moment, he may have wondered if the job was possible as he sputtered "I think I can." He never gave up. As he reached the peak and descended the slope, he exclaimed in fast tempo "I thought I could, I thought I could, I thought I could."

The story shows what we can accomplished when we believe in ourselves. In a world of constant diets and food temptations, the narrative reminds us of what self-encouragement achieves. Like the little engine, we may struggle. Previous attempts may have failed, but we keep going. How close have we come to our goal and decided it was just too much? Faith wavered. We hit a weight plateau, snorted and strained, and wanted to quit. All the effort in the world may have seemed futile.

That little choo-choo has a message for us. He believed success was within reach What is more helpful than to repeat to ourselves "I think l can"? But a word of warning. As the little engine flew down the mountainside, he did not disregard caution. He stayed on track. Often, we reach our weight-loss goal and disregard restraint.

The Apostle Paul endured many obstacles in his ministry. Did he ever feel like giving up? He said, "I can do all things through Christ who strengthens me" (Philippians 4:13 NKJV). By himself, regardless of a positive approach, he understood his inability to accomplish his task without God's help.

God assures us all things are possible with him. Not only can he help us reach our goal, but he can help us remain on track once we have succeeded. Attitude is a potent motivator.

Prayer with Purpose:

Lord, when all around me seems bleak and I'm discouraged in efforts to lose weight, help me remember all things are possible with you. Your encouraging promise is all I need. Amen.

Thoughts to Ponder:

- Negative thoughts produce negative actions.
- Self-encouragement has a powerful influence on what we accomplish.

Lesson for Life:

We can do all things when God gives us the strength and ability.

Digging Deeper

1. Why is self-confidence significant when it comes to losing weight?

____

____

____

____

____

2. When have you reacted as *The Little Engine that Could* in maintaining an appropriate weight?

____

____

____

____

____

3. If God's choice is for you to delay weight loss despite eating a healthy diet, how will you respond?

____

____

____

____

____

19 Pursue Kindness

Kind words are like honey— sweet to the soul and healthy for the body.
Proverbs 16:24

Bitter cold winds defied me to remain upright as I struggled toward the office door. I managed to maneuver my books and bag to let myself in, and I immediately saw Jean. She started toward me with a cup of hot coffee and a cheerful smile. As she offered me the steaming brew, she reached to relieve my loaded arms while I wriggled from my wraps.

"Here, this coffee will warm you and do a body good." The drink didn't warm me nearly as much as her gracious smile and genuine greeting on this horrific winter day. It reminded me of Proverbs 16:24. Kind words are sweet and a proven health benefit. They are pleasant and wholesome and rejuvenate our bodies and souls.

On that morning, weather caused my immediate problems, but soon those challenges would dissipate into more pleasant days. On other occasions, I seemed helpless to conquer my personal struggles or lingering dread, including that shocking number facing me on the scale. We may or may not have an encouraging friend like Jean, but there is Someone who will always be there.

Words of encouragement when we face setbacks at losing weight are like that cup of hot coffee from my coworker. They soothe the chill of our souls in the bitter pangs of defeat. Sometimes friends unintentionally let us down, but God never does.

The songwriter, Arthur A. Luther, penned the words to "Jesus Never Fails." He understood that friends may prove untrue, but Jesus loves and cares for us. The Lord never fails. Even in the midst of life's darkest hour, we can trust his everlasting power and remember his promise.

When we awaken each morning, God knows what our day will be like. He made this day for us to show his compassion through our actions. His presence and love will guide us through whatever comes our way, including what we eat and how we care for our bodies. Days may seem bleak and life pressed down, but what better way to start each day than to remember God has kept us through the night? What greater form of encouragement exists than the Lord's thoughtfulness to us, day in and day out?

How do we best respond toward his kindness? The prophet Isaiah said, "I will mention the loving kindnesses of the LORD And the praises of the LORD, According to all that the LORD has bestowed on us. . . According to the multitude of His loving kindnesses" (Isaiah 63:7 NKJV). Whatever sins or mistakes we make, even eating less-healthy foods, the situation could be worse without God's kindheartedness. He is our inexhaustible fountain of mercy and grace. "Everything he does reveals his glory and majesty. His righteousness never fails" (Psalm 111:3).

Prayer with Purpose:

Dear Lord, keep me mindful of those helpful friends who encourage me through their kind words and deeds. Help me to remember the best friend I have is Jesus. He never fails me. Amen.

Thoughts to Ponder:

- Those who encourage us soothe our souls like a cup of hot coffee warms our bodies on a cold winter day.
- When all others fail us, Jesus never does.
- Thank God for his kindness as he directs our day toward healthy eating.

Lesson for Life:

Friends who encourage us by words or deeds exemplify God's kindness in every aspect of our lives, even in the foods we eat.

Digging Deeper

1. When have you experienced kindness from another and felt that God had placed that person along your path?

____
____
____
____
____

2. When have you allowed God to use you to exhibit his kindness toward others?

____
____
____
____
____

20 Request Help

Why spend your money on food that does you no good? Listen to me, and you will eat what is good. You will enjoy the finest food. . . . Seek the LORD while you can find him. Call on him now while he is near.
Isaiah 55:2,6

Jean Nidetch sought to hide her eating obsession around family and friends. While pretending to resist large quantities of food, she squirreled away cookies. When alone, she sneaked her hidden treasures and gorged herself until stuffed. Her weight soared to 214 pounds, and with a 44-inch waist, danger lurked.

Discouraged by lack of success, she attended a free diet clinic offered by the Board of Health in her city where she successfully lost 20 pounds. Then, her motivation waned. In 1961, Jean recognized she would never break her habit by herself. She called several friends and sought their help. Through confession and support from like-sufferers, she came to realize the significance of sharing her battle with others who were also struggling. The idea of a small group of friends meeting weekly caught on. Other small groups formed to discuss their plight. Two years from that fateful day of contacting friends for help, Jean formed Weight

Watchers, and as men and women worldwide now realize, the rest was history.

Weight Watchers International, Inc. (rebranded in 2018 to WW International, Inc.© to reflect a focus on "Wellness that Works") has proven successful to many where other diets or plans have failed. Much of their success is attributed to the formation of support groups which arm members with the tools and knowledge to succeed (See Choosing a Weight Loss Diet Appendix 11).

How many diets have we started and stopped? Unsound diets are destined for failure from the beginning. They may call for unavailable foods or too many selections we can't prepare or don't like. Prepared diet foods offered by some diet programs can become a financial burden.

How can we succeed? Friends can be helpful as partners and encouragers. What do we do when it is just us and fast-food places or cookies at the office? At times, we falter and eat less-nutritious fares. As Isaiah said, why do we spend money on food that isn't good for us? But Isaiah doesn't leave us there. He says that God will give us his unfailing love. All we need do is seek him.

Maintaining a diet to lose weight isn't easy. It requires determination and commitment most of us don't have. That doesn't mean we are failures—only that we are human. Even when we can't have an encouraging friend or a group with us, we always have God. When we seek him, he is there. It's time to stop and realize he is continually beside us.

Prayer with Purpose:

Lord, may I always seek you in the small as well as in the major areas of life. Guide my decisions, even in foods I eat, and help me to realize you are always with me. Amen.

Thoughts to Ponder:

- Money spent for unhealthy foods can be better used for nourishing ones.
- God wants us to pursue those who will encourage us.
- When we try to make wise food choices, God will help when we ask.

Lesson for Life:

When we seek God, we will find him.

Digging Deeper

1. If you have friends with mutual weight problems and goals, how can you initiate meeting together to seek God in efforts to eat healthy?

____

____

____

____

____

21

Listen

"Go out and stand before me on the mountain," the LORD told him . . . and a mighty windstorm hit the mountain. It was such a terrible blast that the rocks were torn loose, but the LORD was not in the wind. After the wind there was an earthquake, but the LORD was not in the earthquake. And after the earthquake there was a fire, but the LORD was not in the fire. And after the fire there was the sound of a gentle whisper.
1 Kings 19:11-12

Elijah is one of the most recognized prophets in the Old Testament. He is only one of two individuals identified as going directly to heaven from earth without experiencing death. But he, like us, was human. Although he possessed an unsurpassed powerful faith, he had weaknesses. Elijah defied 450 prophets of Baal, yet when threatened by Jezebel, he succumbed to fear. He fled for his life and ended up hiding in a cave on Mt. Sinai (1 Kings 18:21-19:12).

This bold man of God melted into a pity-party before the Lord. He had done all he could, and now he felt alone and dejected, not unlike many of us as we struggle to eat right. We think we do all the right things yet fail to reduce weight. The Lord would have none of Elijah's whining. With all Elijah had achieved, he failed to look to God in his time of vulnerability. God unleashed his power in windstorms, earthquakes, and fire. But the Holy One was not present in any of these. God spoke to Elijah in a gentle whisper.

How does God speak to us? Do we often expect some spectacular dramatization from God when we feel beaten down and defeated? Just as Elijah needed to listen to the soft calling of the Lord, so do we. God may speak to us quietly at unexpected times as he tries to teach us to rely on him. Imagine the difference we could make in our eating habits if we seek him before stuffing ourselves with food (See Tips for Cutting Calories Appendix 12).

It isn't easy to rely on God. We become distracted with life. We believe we should be able to accomplish tasks all by ourselves. God understands as he waits for us to pay attention. Several verses in the Scriptures talk about God's response. He listens and wants to meet our needs when we serve him in accordance with his will.

The Gospel of Mark relates Jesus' response. "I tell you, you can pray for anything, and if you believe that you've received it, it will be yours" (Mark 11:24).

John 16:23-24 also gives an account of Jesus' words to his disciples. "At that time you won't need to ask me for anything. I tell you the truth, you will ask the Father directly, and he will grant your request because you use my name. . . . Ask, using my name, and you will receive, and you will have abundant joy."

When will we listen to his words? While God speaks to us and answers our prayers, his response isn't always what we expect. We may not lose that excess fat immediately. He may want to teach us patience, humility, or reliance on him as pounds fail to drop off. Whatever his answer and message—listen.

Prayer with Purpose:

Lord, teach me to listen and hear your will so that I may make healthier choices in foods I eat. Amen.

Thoughts to Ponder:

- Like Elijah who had faith and many strengths, we all have weaknesses.
- God doesn't need to shout for us to hear him.
- Asking God to increase our faith and help us stay more disciplined in our eating choices improves our chances of losing weight.
- The practice of prayer perfects our listening skills.

Lesson for Life:

Listening to God's whispers triumphs over the shout of crowds.

Digging Deeper

1. How will you improve your listening skills to hear what God has to say to you?

____
____
____
____
____

2. Share times when God's whispers revealed to you his omnipotence and desires for you.

____
____
____
____
____

3. Did any of those occasions relate to food?

____
____
____
____
____

Part IV
God's Promises

22

Eternal Blessing

Remember, it is sin to know what you ought to do and then not do it. James 4:17

In biblical times, the first-born male acquired a special blessing and most of his father's inheritance. When Jacob and Esau were born, Esau arrived first, but Jacob came quickly behind with his hand on Esau's heel (Genesis 25:25-26).

Jacob was a deceiver, as his name implied. Sure, his mother favored him and could have been part of the problem. But his brother Esau had troubles, too. He seemed more concerned with immediate pleasure and satisfaction than future assurances of God. He did the unthinkable and gave away his guaranteed promise in exchange for food (Genesis 25:29-34). Yes, at the time he was hungry, but to let food and immediate desires become more important than God's blessing was nothing less than a travesty.

Esau, an avid hunter, prepared dishes made from wild game. Returning from one of his adventures, evidently empty handed, he longed for a good meal. Jacob had prepared a red stew, probably made from lentils or grains. Esau couldn't resist. He asked for a portion.

Scriptures seem to omit a lot of conversation between these twins. When Esau requested the stew, Jacob, the second born of Isaac, connived to take the blessing of his father from Esau. He took advantage of his brother's craving for food and required Esau to swear an oath relinquishing his birthright and pledge from God. We have no indication Esau hesitated. It's unlikely he was to the point of starvation, but at that moment, a full stomach became more important than the priceless birthright. Esau despised his birthright and willingly exchanged it for food. "Look, I'm dying of starvation!" said Esau. "What good is my birthright to me now?" (Genesis 25:32).

Whether right or wrong, Jacob seized the opportunity. Whatever way we interpret this story, the initial fault lay with Esau. He gave away something irreplaceable in return for the satisfaction of a little stew. He would be hungry again, but he would never have the opportunity to regain his birthright.

Often, we may carelessly respond like Esau. What are we exchanging for the temptations of sweet, rich foods? We are hungry, and time and again we eat less-nourishing foods and compromise our health. We grab fast food or unhealthy snacks because of a slight hunger pang.

When was the last time we ate something we knew wasn't the best choice for a healthy weight or lifestyle? It's doubtful we sacrificed anything material or a special blessing. But we may have willingly given up long-term goals to choose healthy fares to indulge in short-term decadent pleasures. Our downfall may have resulted from a lapse in judgment. Eating a plate of fried catfish or French fries and a Big Mac® on occasion probably won't kill us, but if we continue such a pattern of eating, it can interfere with future health (See Tips for Eating Out Appendix 13).

We don't see in this biblical example of Jacob and Esau that either sought God's will. Each one knew what he wanted. For

Esau at that moment, food was all he could think of. We don't know the inward character of Esau except he was impatient and sought immediate gratification even when it meant a permanent sacrifice. As for Jacob, he was a schemer who tricked his brother into giving up his birthright, and more importantly, God's promised blessing. While Jacob was less than perfect, he found favor with God. Perhaps because he recognized God's omnipotence and understood the long-term benefits.

When we reflect on our inner character, what do we see? Are we impulsive and seek instant rewards from food? What extended blessings have we traded for immediate gratification?

Prayer with Purpose:

Lord, thank you for the blessings you constantly provide. Help me avoid giving in to hunger attacks that may compromise blessings you have promised. Amen.

Thoughts to Ponder:

- When we know the right choices to make and fail to do so, what we do is wrong.
- Exchanging unhealthy snacks for a reprieve from hunger may have immediate or lasting health consequences.

Lesson for Life:

Spontaneous unhealthy eating may jeopardize future blessings of good health.

Digging Deeper

1. Scripture says if we know what we are doing is wrong, it is sin. Do you ever consider what you eat as sinful?

____

____

____

____

____

2. How can you cease to eat unhealthy foods in order to receive God's blessing of better health?

____

____

____

____

____

23

Answered Prayer

Pray for each other. . . . The earnest prayer of a righteous person has great power and produces wonderful results.
James 5:16

When our younger daughter finished high school, she had a chance to travel abroad with a choral group. I wanted her to take advantage of the opportunity, but she was headed to college that fall, and we couldn't afford both. The trip cost about $1,000, a lot of money at the time. She, too, knew funds were needed for college expenses. What should she do? I reassured her that if we prayed, God would help her find an answer—whether yes or no.

"But my sister has a $1,000 insurance policy made to me. I'm afraid if I pray for the money, something may happen to her."

That thought never entered my mind, but she was anxious. She sought to figure out in human terms how God would provide. Her concern was misguided. When we pray, putting God's will first is a priority as we realize his answers aren't always the responses we seek. However, my daughter and I prayed that no harm would come to her sister.

A few weeks later she called. "I won the writing contest I entered last spring, and they have awarded me $1,000."

Months earlier she had entered the contest promoted by a civic organization. I never thought about the contest and don't think she had either. But God didn't forget. He honored her prayer with the exact amount of money she needed. Had my daughter failed to enter the contest, she wouldn't have won the prize. When we do our part, God provides what we need even when we fail to see a way. And nothing bad happened to her sister.

Now will praying make us thinner? What are we doing to lose weight and enjoy better health? Several friends who have struggled for many years with weight issues have shared how their outlook and size altered when they finally relinquished control of their situation to God. They stopped placing emphasis on feeble efforts to control their weight and sought God to help them choose foods wisely and allow him to take charge of the calorie counting.

There's something to be said for attempting to do all we can. But we need God's help to succeed. His power working through us will more readily help us reach a healthy goal.

Prayer with Purpose:

Lord, when I fail to lose pounds through my efforts, remind me to keep my focus on you instead of my continuing failure. May I commune with you more faithfully and rely on your will for my body size. Amen.

Thoughts to Ponder:

- Our prayers and those of others can have unbelievable results.
- We can be the size and weight God wants when we relinquish our eating problems to him.
- God answers prayers in his way, not ours.

Lesson for Life:

Faith in God yields more positive results than focus on self.

Digging Deeper

1. When have you made food choices and weight loss a matter of prayer?

____

____

____

____

____

2. What leads you to believe God does or does not answer your prayers?

____

____

____

____

____

24 Followed Convictions

But if you have doubts about whether or not you should eat something, you are sinning if you go ahead and do it. For you are not following your convictions. If you do anything you believe is not right, you are sinning.
Romans 14:23

My mother reared my much older siblings during the Great Depression. Her frugality of those years carried over into the rationings during World War II. Experiences made her mindful of each penny she spent. Once when shopping, we became thirsty. When I mentioned getting a cola, she said thoughtfully, "That's five-cents I can save to buy something else."

By no means was she selfish or stingy. Her generosity exceeded that of many well-to-do matrons. But I learned a valuable lesson from her use of money. She made choices based on what was more important. Was she so thirsty she could not wait until we were home to get something to drink? That nickel was a lot of money in terms of food and clothing she needed to buy. She was willing to relinquish a brief whim for greater priorities.

As an adult, I understand how her lesson applied in many areas, especially in my outlook on health. What if we stopped to consider those same results when it comes to calories in food?

All too often we succumb to self-indulgent pleasures. Any food with carbohydrates, fats, or proteins has calories essential for energy (See Nutrients for Good Health Appendix 14). When we consume more calories than our bodies need, they are stored as fat and cause our physique to increase in size. We know only too well that extra calories pack themselves onto our hips or elsewhere. It's all about choice.

Regular Coca Cola, for example, contains about 100 calories per eight ounces. Theoretically, we must walk about one mile to burn those 100 calories. Now the choice is ours. Are we willing to walk an additional mile to get rid of those extra calories? Just as my mother gave up a bottled drink to buy something more essential, will we choose 100 empty calories or select something more nutritious? Giving up added snacks or higher calorie foods will help avoid excess body fat. Can we decide, like my mother, to skip the cola and spend valuable nutrient-dense calories on foods that will result in better health?

Maybe we should stop and compare all those additional calories to harmful financial situations. If we selectively buy needed items instead of wasting money on frivolous things, our cash seems to stretch farther. When we limit empty calories, we have more to invest in better choices. With God's help, we can make every calorie count.

Prayer with Purpose:

Lord, help me choose foods which provide nourishment for my body and to avoid those that will only add additional body fat. Amen.

Thoughts to Ponder:

- Carbohydrates, fats, and proteins are our only food sources of calories.
- Choosing lower-calorie nutritious foods instead of empty calories helps maintain control of our weight.
- In our society, we are unlikely to suffer health consequences from brief hunger pangs.

Lesson for Life:

Eating empty calories is like putting counterfeit money into a bank account.

Digging Deeper

1. What are your personal convictions about losing weight?

____
____
____
____
____

2. What simple changes can you make in your eating habits that will lower the number of calories you eat?

____
____
____
____
____

25

Strength from God's Grace

Jesus Christ is the same yesterday, today, and forever. So do not be attracted by strange, new ideas. Your strength comes from God's grace, not from rules about food, which don't help those who follow them.
Hebrews 13:8-9

A friend stopped by our home unexpectedly. As soon as he entered, I sensed something was wrong. As the story unfolded, he had made a grievous financial error—more correctly an addiction error. The previous night, he had gone on a gambling spree, lost all his savings, and written hot checks on his account. He made a mistake, and now he faced the consequences. Through the next several months, we worked with him to get his finances and life back in order.

Everyone makes mistakes. Some results are costly, whether financial or otherwise. Many prove embarrassing, others just inconvenient. What is significant is whether we own up to our responsibilities and confront the results. Trusted friends may help us see solutions we haven't considered. One thing is sure, God promised to always be with us. The writer of Hebrews said, "For God has said, 'I will never fail you. I will never abandon you.' So we can say with confidence, 'The LORD is my helper, so I will have no fear'" (Hebrews 13:5-6).

Once we overindulge in food, we face consequences. If we believe we are plagued with overeating and weight issues we can't resolve and the scales confirm the situation, how will we correct the problem? Do we take blame when we are the reason for our own weight crisis? Do we need to do something about it? For multiple reasons, yes.

Like our friend with his gambling addiction, the first step to recovery is to admit to ourselves and close friends that we have a growing dilemma. None of us can wish we were smaller, and it suddenly happens. We can't go to bed and awaken the next morning five, ten, twenty-five, or fifty pounds lighter. So, what is the solution?

When we discuss this issue with God, we learn a different perspective. Communication with him isn't some simple "Oh, God make me thin." It's a heart-felt plea for God to come alongside and help. That aid may come in the form of a friend who lovingly guides and encourages us toward healthier foods. Or our prayer time with God may imbue us with the confidence and desire to exchange less-healthy fares for nutritious, lower-calorie options. Perhaps the Holy Spirit will convict us to avoid the latest food fad.

The writer of Hebrews also warns against attraction to new ideas. Sometimes we're gullible like our addicted gambling friend and yield to the latest diet craze. Food rules set by those who focus on emptying our pockets instead of improving our health are a scourge to the dieter. Story after story recounts the deadly consequences of popular but dangerous supplements. The wise avoids strange new diet ideas or trying unknown supplement sources. It's smart to be leery of promises made without substantial credibility. God can and does allow our paths to cross with those who give reliable information and seek our best interest for better health.

Let's not overlook the greatest source available. There's hope beyond diets and exercise. The Holy Spirit intercedes to God on our behalf when we pray for control over our eating habits. God is our all-sufficient help. His grace strengthens us to make wiser food choices. Without him we can't do anything, but with him, all things are possible.

Prayer with Purpose:

Lord, remind me that even small adjustments in what I choose to eat can help me reach a healthier weight. Please guide me to remember and make changes that will keep me more physically fit. Thank you, God, for always being available to aid me. Amen.

Thoughts to Ponder:

- God wants to be our number one partner for healthy eating.
- "New idea" diets may prove useless or sometimes dangerous.
- Trusted friends who encourage us can make our weight problems easier.

Lesson for Life:

God will join us in our efforts to improve our eating choices.

Digging Deeper

1. How do you interpret "Your strength comes from God's grace, not from rules about food"? What are your personal convictions about losing weight?

26 Positive Expectations

God will make this happen, for he who calls you is faithful. 1 Thessalonians 5:24

I had purchased several pieces of furniture while visiting in another state. The company assured me they would ship them immediately. Six weeks passed. During that period, the store sent five electronic notices moving the shipping date farther out. When they called to inform me it would arrive in a four-hour window on week eight, it was a day I had previous commitments I could not change. I offered the day before or the day after. They would not budge and expressed no concern for the long wait or inconvenience. My thoughts shifted from disappointment to anger. I could feel my body become tense and my heart rate increase. A positive attitude eluded me.

When expectations aren't met, whether for purchases or for losing weight, we feel disillusioned, defeated, and resentful. Have we lost all hope of getting rid of those bulges we consider unsightly? When the digital number on our scale seems stuck, we may feel abandoned, forsaken.

I was unhappy about a delayed furniture shipment and the hassle it caused. It became a case of persistence in hounding the company's shipping department. Are we as dogged about weight-loss as I was about getting that furniture? More importantly, how is our extra weight affecting our health? Do we think God has abandoned us when excess fat lingers on our bodies? Does he care?

God knows our needs and our distress. We can regain hope. He will help us on his timeline. The psalmist reminded us to "give [our] burdens to the Lord, and he will take care of [us]" (Psalm 55:22). The disciple Peter repeats this message, "Give all your worries and cares to God, for he cares about you" (1 Peter 5:7). Do we believe that?

What would change if we spent more time talking with God than in eating? I suspect many of us think more about food or the weight we want to lose than our relationship with a Heavenly Father. We aren't saddled with a negative God who has no interest in our weight problems but with one who accents positives. When we concentrate more on him and less on ourselves, the focus of our lives changes. With spiritual changes may come physical changes. If we are doing our part, the final decision is up to our Lord. Do we have the faith to trust him in all things, even to how much he wants us to weigh?

Prayer with Purpose:

Lord, help me to talk with you more and think about food less. May I make efforts to eat a healthier diet and then rely on you for positive results. Amen.

Thoughts to Ponder:

- When we feel distraught and don't know where to turn next, we can seek God's positive reinforcement.
- God can take our negatives and turn them into positives.

Lesson for Life:

As we talk to God more, he keeps us positive about ourselves in the face of negatives.

Digging Deeper

1. What steps can and will you take to develop a healthy and positive attitude toward food?

____

____

____

____

____

2. How will you seek to improve all your communication with God?

____

____

____

____

____

27

Fickle Scale—Faithful God

Great is his faithfulness; his mercies begin afresh each morning.
Lamentations 3:23

I stepped on the scale and glared at the number. It showed I was barely an appropriate weight for my height. Always weight conscious, but never inclined to diet or make a big fuss, I decided it would be great to lose ten pounds. Without much fanfare or commitment, I continued to eat basically the same diet while watching and limiting excessive sweets. About a year later, my scale had gone berserk. The digital dial had moved in the wrong direction. Instead of losing the desired weight, much to my horror, the number increased ten pounds. What happened? My endocrinologist had shifted a medication I knew could make a difference in weight. Complaints to her fell on deaf ears.

The extra weight had consequences. Clothes became tighter. I needed a new wardrobe. My attitude changed. What happened to that skinny person I used to be? Discouraged? Yes. Did God care about such mundane things as a little too much weight? After all, through appropriate health care, I could function. How could I possibly complain? God blessed me with many years, despite multiple health issues. However, I wasn't happy with those additional pounds. With age creeping upward, metabolism slows while ailments treated by medications that affect weight may increase (See Common Medications and Weight Gain Appendix 15). Millions face the same dilemma—those formerly an appropriate weight now weigh too much.

The prophet Jeremiah faced numerous obstacles much more significant than a little extra weight. In Lamentations, he bemoaned the fate resulting from God's anger. He believed God had "besieged and surrounded [him] with anguish and distress" (Lamentations 3:5). God had buried him in a dark place, walled in, and he could not escape (Lamentations 3:6-7). The Lord even seemed to shut out his prayers (Lamentations 3:7).

We too may feel under siege like Jeremiah. God may not be angry, but we may sometimes think our prayers about losing weight go unanswered. Eventually, Jeremiah had hope and proclaimed, "The faithful love of the Lord never ends. Great is his faithfulness" (Lamentations 3:23). We too can have hope because God is faithful.

Scales may appear fickle when higher weight shows than we believe it should be, but God always blesses us. He is faithful even when scales and weight are inconsistent. "The LORD is good to those who depend on him, to those who search for him" (Lamentations 3:25).

Prayer with Purpose:

God, we are blessed with medical care to keep us well, even when it may cause us to gain weight. Help us to count those blessings you give daily and to rely on your everlasting faithfulness. Amen.

Thoughts to Ponder:

- Some medications can cause weight gain.
- Everyone's metabolism decreases with age resulting in greater probability of weight gain.
- To keep the weight of younger years requires more exercise and fewer calories.
- God is faithful even in our distress.

Lesson for Life:

God is faithful when everything around us seems inconsistent.

Digging Deeper

1. When have you assessed your weight gain through appropriate medical testing and medications?

____

____

____

____

____

2. How can you express your gratitude to God for the health you do have, and what are you willing to do to stay healthy?

____

____

____

____

____

28 Never Deserted

What's more, I am with you, and I will protect you wherever you go. One day I will bring you back to this land. I will not leave you until I have finished giving you everything I have promised you. Genesis 28:15

The biblical story of Job tells of a godly man who lost all his children and worldly possessions. Not only that, he experienced failing health and a body covered with sores. What purpose did his life have? He questioned why God allowed him to live. If he had died at birth, he would have peace (Job 3:11-13). Do we ever feel like Job?

Job felt God had deserted him. God had struck him down and his terror fought against him (Job 6:4). Job felt he had every right to complain (Job 6:5). He reminded God how people whine about unsalted food and tasteless egg whites (Job 6:6). The distress even took Job's appetite (Job 6:4-7).

Unwise diet plans may become tiresome, tasteless, and boring. We can't stand them for long and have no appetite for them. At this point, we often cave in for more delectable foods that sabotage our efforts at healthy eating. Do we sometime feel we have every right to grumble about our plight of too much weight?

Regardless of our situations, God understands. Nothing is hidden from him. As Solomon's father pointed out to him, "Serve [God] with a perfect heart and with a willing mind: for the Lord searcheth all hearts and understandeth all the imaginations of the thoughts" (1 Chronicles 28:9 KJV). We would do well to remember that. God knows what is in our hearts, every thought even before we think it.

Do we allow him to constantly lead the way even as we determine what we will put into our mouths? What if we started each day with the thought that we will seek his help in every bite we take? Would it change the focus of our day and our diet? In his infinite mercy, God gives us peace about weight and diet. "'For the mountains may depart and the hills disappear, but my kindness shall not leave you. My promise of peace for you will never be broken,' says the Lord who has mercy upon [us]" (Isaiah 54:10 TLB). God never deserts his own, whatever obstacles we face in changing to healthier eating habits. He protects and will never leave us.

Prayer with Purpose:

Lord, I become tired and bored with endless dieting. Renew my spirit to choose healthy foods, put fad diets aside, and allow you to work in my life. Amen.

Thoughts to Ponder:

- Endless fad diets become boring and tedious to follow.
- God cares what we eat each day.
- God is always available and will guide us to make wise food choices.

Lesson for Life:

Fad diets or quick weight-loss plans cannot replace God's wisdom working through us to choose healthy foods.

Digging Deeper

1. Do you ever feel deserted in your struggle to lose weight?

2. If so, how can you benefit from Job's words found in today's devotional?

3. What is your usual response when you become bored with varied diets?

4. How can you break your habit of following the current fad diet and adhere to one that is wholesome?

____

____

____

____

____

PART V
God's Will

29 Bearing Accountability

O LORD, who are we that you should notice us, mere mortals that you should care for us? Psalm 144:3

I live in a beautiful neighborhood. In certain areas, homeowners have problems with drainage. Occasionally, neighbors in those sections experience difficulties because they neglected areas near the lake or ditches unaware it was part of their property. They believed the problem should be attended by their homeowners' association or the city. As an association board member, it's difficult to clarify how unintentional neglect of overgrown grass, weeds, and accumulation of brush resulted in major drainage issues. Their disregard made remedy more difficult and expensive to correct. Although many thought otherwise, it was their problem to fix because it was their property.

When it comes to issues with our bodies, we may have ignored preventive healthcare, and now conditions have resulted which may not heal easily, if at all. We blame the food industry for sugary drinks or fatty foods that cause problems. Some of us blame technology or entertainment for sedentary lifestyles. We fault physicians and health care workers for their inability to cure diseases caused by smoking, overeating, or other poor health habits.

It's always someone else's fault. We hold them responsible for problems due to our own negligence or failure to accept responsibility for our health. Sometimes, we blame God. He gave us this body, and we think he should keep it well even when we choose to abuse it.

Our earthly bodies were not made to last forever but, "We never give up. Though our bodies are dying, our spirits are being renewed every day" (2 Corinthians 4:16). However, what we eat will make a difference (See Seven Principles for a Healthier Diet Appendix 16).

Those homeowners felt someone else was responsible for their property maintenance. We may think the same way. Who have we blamed or felt responsible for the excess weight on our bodies? When we take accountability for our choices, we avert many physical problems. It's up to us to put healthy foods and appropriate calories into our bodies. What are we doing to protect them?

Prayer with Purpose:

Lord, help me to realize this body you gave me is my responsibility. Help me to treat it kindly with healthy foods and proper care. Amen.

Thoughts to Ponder:

- Unintended neglect doesn't excuse physical problems resulting from excessive weight.
- Care for our bodies is our responsibility.
- Reliable resources are available when we don't know how or what to choose for healthy eating.

Lesson for Life:

Our bodies require appropriate care to function properly.

Digging Deeper

1. If you assessed your everyday situation, would you classify yourself as obedient or stubborn to health needs?

____

____

____

____

____

2. Are you a risk-taker, willing to risk your health by eating whatever you want whether it is healthy or not?

____

____

____

____

____

3. Your body is your obligation. How will you take responsibility in the future for your physical well-being by choosing to eat foods to maintain your health and an appropriate weight?

____

____

____

____

____

30

Focus to Win

I focus on this one thing: Forgetting the past and looking forward to what lies ahead, I press on to reach the end of the race and receive the heavenly prize for which God, through Christ Jesus, is calling us.
Philippians 3:13-14

An Olympic skier with a gold metal within her grasp looked back to check her competition as she neared the finish line. In that split second, this obvious winner slipped and fell. With success in sight, her lapse of focus cost a gold medal.

Our desired weight-goal may be within reach, but if we lose focus and fall prey to oppositions, we may fail to reach that finish line. Too often we reflect on the past without looking forward. Negative thoughts creep in. Doubts surface. We recall how often losing weight or keeping it off escaped us. Why try one more time? We're convinced we will only fail again—and again. We allow ourselves to linger in the presence of tempting foods too difficult to resist. One split second of yielding to temptations sets up a scenario to fail to reach that finish line. My friend who has struggled a lifetime with weight issues said, "I had to respond differently to tempting foods and remember what I wanted long term while working in the short term." She understood the significance to remain focused.

Our morale, not to mention our faith, is at its lowest ebb. Past failures become an excuse to stop trying. Why have we failed? Each of us may have a different reason or excuse. Is our thinking accurate? Why have we failed? My friend said, "More often past failures have the ability to profoundly discourage us. We actually begin to believe that weight loss isn't possible for us."

Occasionally we hear of heroic physically challenged persons who enter a marathon they can't possibly win. Yet, they persist, and as they cross the finish line in spite of difficulty, the crowds cheer—not because of winning, but because of perseverance. Why can't we be as diligent as these determined people?

Paul said he focused on one thing—winning the prize before him. Do we? Do we remain focused until we attain our desired goal?

Prayer with Purpose:

Lord, you alone can keep me focused. Restrain me from looking back at failures and help me to press on. Amen.

Thoughts to Ponder:

- Looking back may cause us to lose the "weight loss race" instead of winning.
- The more we press on, the sooner our goal comes into sight.
- God desires for us to win the race against overweight and obesity.

Lesson for Life:

Focus is a discipline that helps us win the prize.

Digging Deeper

1. It is a natural characteristic to want to win, regardless of the competition or the situation. God wants you to win the race in your personal "battle of the bulge." He wants you to be a healthy weight in order to accomplish what he desires for you to do. What steps will you take in the future to assure that you will do your part in seeking to become and maintain a healthy weight?

____

____

____

____

____

31 God's Masterpiece

For we are God's masterpiece. He has created us anew in Christ Jesus, so we can do the good things he planned for us long ago.
Ephesians 2:10

When our daughter travels through European cities, she enjoys visiting well-known museums and places of art. She appreciates the fine paintings and sculptures of renowned artists. Not all of us understand or value the nuances of the skilled hand strokes that become priceless works. However, we do recognize efforts and beauty by their creators.

One of the most renowned paintings of all time is Michelangelo's biblical portrayals on the ceiling of the Sistine Chapel. His frescos are unsurpassed. Michelangelo created this masterpiece even though he considered himself a sculptor, not a painter.

When God formed each of us, he created unique individuals. The most skilled artist created us and called us his masterpieces. Can we imagine? We may not perceive ourselves as works of art. As Michelangelo could not see himself a painter, we may fail to envision ourselves as beautiful vessels. But God sees each of us as a magnificent treasure. Or we may feel like a friend of mine. "I know spiritually I am a masterpiece, but as an overweight person I struggle to see my body as a masterpiece." Dear friends, God sees every part of us as a masterpiece, both physically and spiritually.

Maybe we do strive to take care of God's work of art, but the pounds stay put. Whatever our weight status, God points to us as examples of his grace and kindness for future generations (Ephesians 2:7).

Have we carefully cared for our human work of art so the beauty he created is preserved? Do we know where to find reliable information for healthy eating (See Reliable Internet Links Appendix 17)? What will we do from this point forward to make wise choices to care for his splendid structures?

Choices throughout our lifetimes can mar or preserve his masterpieces. God is rich in mercy, even when we make a wreck of our lives or fail to follow habits that glorify him. When we look at our reflections, may we remember the value God has placed on each of us.

Prayer with Purpose:

Lord, keep me mindful that you consider me one of your masterpieces. Help me to care for this precious gift in all that I do, especially the foods I eat. Amen.

Thoughts to Ponder:

- We become God's masterpieces of grace when we are created anew through Christ Jesus.
- God fashioned us as his masterpieces so we could do the good things he planned for us.
- Artists seek to protect their work from damage. Should we do less in the care of our bodies?

Lesson for Life:

Regardless of background or physical well-being, God created each of us as a masterpiece.

Digging Deeper

1. You are God's magnificent creation—whatever your size, ethnic origin, physical appearance, or any of the many traits humans use to judge each other. Knowing that you are God's special handiwork, how do you assess the features and physical attributes he has given you?

____

____

____

____

____

2. Do you make every effort to keep your body healthy and well?

____

____

____

____

____

3. Do you avoid foods and environmental situations that could shorten your lifespan?

____

____

____

____

____

4. Have you placed your complete trust in Jesus to live the life he chooses for you to live?

____

____

____

____

____

5. From this day forward, how will you honor God by honoring the body he has given you?

____

____

____

____

____

Appendices

Appendix 1
Body Mass Index (BMI) Chart[1]

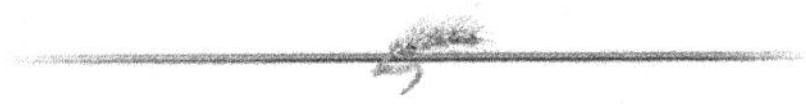

The BMI chart on the next page identifies different weight levels based on height and weight. While it isn't a perfect model, the instrument is an accessible tool to assess appropriate weight.

To check your BMI, on the far-left vertical row, find your height. Move horizontally across the row until you find the weight corresponding closest to your current weight. Move your finger upward to the very top horizontal line above the chart to read your BMI. If your weight and height exceed numbers on this chart (BMI above 35), check the following expanded link to find your BMI.

[1]https://www.nhlbi.nih.gov/health/educational/lose_wt/BMI/bmi_tbl.pdf

Body Mass Index Table

	Normal						Overweight					Obese										Extreme Obesity														
BMI	**19**	**20**	**21**	**22**	**23**	**24**	**25**	**26**	**27**	**28**	**29**	**30**	**31**	**32**	**33**	**34**	**35**	**36**	**37**	**38**	**39**	**40**	**41**	**42**	**43**	**44**	**45**	**46**	**47**	**48**	**49**	**50**	**51**	**52**	**53**	**54**
Height (inches)																**Body Weight (pounds)**																				
58	91	96	100	105	110	115	119	124	129	134	138	143	148	153	158	162	167	172	177	181	186	191	196	201	205	210	215	220	224	229	234	239	244	248	253	258
59	94	99	104	109	114	119	124	128	133	138	143	148	153	158	163	168	173	178	183	188	193	198	203	208	212	217	222	227	232	237	242	247	252	257	262	267
60	97	102	107	112	118	123	128	133	138	143	148	153	158	163	168	174	179	184	189	194	199	204	209	215	220	225	230	235	240	245	250	255	261	266	271	276
61	100	106	111	116	122	127	132	137	143	148	153	158	164	169	174	180	185	190	195	201	206	211	217	222	227	232	238	243	248	254	259	264	269	275	280	285
62	104	109	115	120	126	131	136	142	147	153	158	164	169	175	180	186	191	196	202	207	213	218	224	229	235	240	246	251	256	262	267	273	278	284	289	295
63	107	113	118	124	130	135	141	146	152	158	163	169	175	180	186	191	197	203	208	214	220	225	231	237	242	248	254	259	265	270	278	282	287	293	299	304
64	110	116	122	128	134	140	145	151	157	163	169	174	180	186	192	197	204	209	215	221	227	232	238	244	250	256	262	267	273	279	285	291	296	302	308	314
65	114	120	126	132	138	144	150	156	162	168	174	180	186	192	198	204	210	216	222	228	234	240	246	252	258	264	270	276	282	288	294	300	306	312	318	324
66	118	124	130	136	142	148	155	161	167	173	179	186	192	198	204	210	216	223	229	235	241	247	253	260	266	272	278	284	291	297	303	309	315	322	328	334
67	121	127	134	140	146	153	159	166	172	178	185	191	198	204	211	217	223	230	236	242	249	255	261	268	274	280	287	293	299	306	312	319	325	331	338	344
68	125	131	138	144	151	158	164	171	177	184	190	197	203	210	216	223	230	236	243	249	256	262	269	276	282	289	295	302	308	315	322	328	335	341	348	354
69	128	135	142	149	155	162	169	176	182	189	196	203	209	216	223	230	236	243	250	257	263	270	277	284	291	297	304	311	318	324	331	338	345	351	358	365
70	132	139	146	153	160	167	174	181	188	195	202	209	216	222	229	236	243	250	257	264	271	278	285	292	299	306	313	320	327	334	341	348	355	362	369	376
71	136	143	150	157	165	172	179	186	193	200	208	215	222	229	236	243	250	257	265	272	279	286	293	301	308	315	322	329	338	343	351	358	365	372	379	386
72	140	147	154	162	169	177	184	191	199	206	213	221	228	235	242	250	258	265	272	279	287	294	302	309	316	324	331	338	346	353	361	368	375	383	390	397
73	144	151	159	166	174	182	189	197	204	212	219	227	235	242	250	257	265	272	280	288	295	302	310	318	325	333	340	348	355	363	371	378	386	393	401	408
74	148	155	163	171	179	186	194	202	210	218	225	233	241	249	256	264	272	280	287	295	303	311	319	326	334	342	350	358	365	373	381	389	396	404	412	420
75	152	160	168	176	184	192	200	208	216	224	232	240	248	256	264	272	279	287	295	303	311	319	327	335	343	351	359	367	375	383	391	399	407	415	423	431
76	156	164	172	180	189	197	205	213	221	230	238	246	254	263	271	279	287	295	304	312	320	328	336	344	353	361	369	377	385	394	402	410	418	426	435	443

Source: Adapted from *Clinical Guidelines on the Identification, Evaluation, and Treatment of Overweight and Obesity in Adults: The Evidence Report.*

Appendix 2
Classifications of Obesity[2]

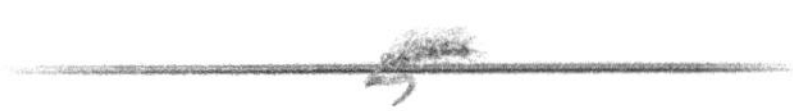

- A BMI < 16 indicates severe thinness
- A BMI 16-17 indicates moderate thinness
- A BMI 17-18.5 indicates mild thinness
- A BMI 18.5-25 indicates normal weight
- A BMI 25-30 indicates overweight
- A BMI 30-35 indicates Class I obesity
- A BMI 35-40 indicates Class II obesity
- A BMI > 40 indicates Class III obesity, sometimes referred to as "extreme" or "severe" obesity

[2]https://www.cdc.gov/obesity/adult/defining.html

Appendix 3

Strategies for Developing a Better Eating Pattern[3]

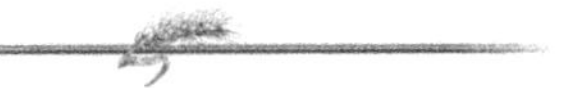

- **Follow a healthy eating pattern.**
  All food and beverage choices matter. Choose a healthy eating pattern at an appropriate calorie level to help achieve and maintain a healthy body weight, support nutrient adequacy, and reduce the risk of chronic disease.

- **Focus on variety, nutrient density, and amount.**
  To meet nutrient needs within calorie limits, choose a variety of nutrient-dense foods across and within all food groups in recommended amounts.

- **Limit calories from added sugars and saturated fats and reduce sodium intake.**
  Cut back on foods and beverages higher in these components to amounts that fit within healthy eating patterns.

- **Shift to healthier food and beverage choices.**
  Choose nutrient-dense foods and beverages within all food groups in place of less healthy choices.

[3]Adapted from: 2015-2020 Dietary Guideline for Americans https://health.gov/dietaryguidelines/2015/guidelines/executive-summary/#key-recs

Appendix 4
Foods to Limit for a Healthy Diet[4]

A healthy eating pattern limits added sugars, saturated fats, trans fats, sodium and alcohol.[2]

Sugars

- Added sugars provide sweetness to improve palatability of foods, help with preservation, and contribute to functional properties such as viscosity, texture, body, color, and browning.
- Many foods with added sugars may contribute to excess calorie intake without contributing to diet quality making it difficult to meet nutritional needs while staying within calorie limits.
- Naturally occurring sugars, such as those in fruit or milk, are not added sugars. Added sugars include brown sugar, corn sweetener, corn syrup, dextrose, fructose, glucose, high-fructose corn syrup, honey, invert sugar, lactose, malt syrup, maltose, molasses, raw sugar, sucrose, trehalose, and turbinado sugar.
- A healthy diet contains less than 10 percent of calories per day from added sugars.
- Questions remain about the effectiveness of high-intensity sweeteners as a long-term weight management strategy. The U.S. Food and Drug Administration (FDA) has approved saccharin, aspartame, acesulfame potassium (Ace-K), and sucralose.

[4]Adapted from 2015-2020 Dietary Guidelines for Americans

FATS, OILS, AND *TRANS* FATS

- Saturated fats, found mostly in animals, are usually solid at room temperature. Main sources in the U.S. diet include mixed dishes containing cheese, meat, or both, such as burgers, sandwiches, and tacos; pizza; rice, pasta, and grain dishes; and meat, poultry, and seafood dishes.
- A healthy diet contains less than 10 percent of calories per day from saturated fats.
- Oils are fats high in monounsaturated and polyunsaturated fats. They are usually liquid at room temperature, and most are derived from plant sources.
- *Trans* fats occur naturally in some foods and are present in small quantities in the cream (fat) of dairy products and meats. They are produced during hydrogenation, a process food manufacturers use to make products with unsaturated fatty acids solid at room temperature. Partial hydrogenation converts unsaturated fatty acids to saturated fatty acids. They are found in some processed foods, i.e. desserts, microwave popcorn, frozen pizza, margarines, and coffee creamers. Increased intake of trans fats elevates LDL cholesterol and raises risks of cardiovascular disease.

SODIUM

- Sodium, primarily consumed as salt (sodium chloride), is an essential nutrient needed by the body in relatively small quantities. Salt is used in curing meat, baking, thickening, enhancing flavor, as a preservative, and in retaining moisture. Food products with salt include mixed dishes such as burgers, sandwiches, and tacos; rice, pasta, and grain dishes; pizza; meat, poultry, and seafood dishes; and soups.

- Health professionals recommend less than 2,300 mg of sodium per day for adults and children ages 14 years and older.

- Recommended levels for individuals with hypertension and pre-hypertension are 1,500 mg per day.

Alcohol

- If alcohol is consumed, it should be in moderation—up to one drink per day for women and up to two drinks per day for men—and only by adults of legal drinking age.

Appendix 5
Healthy Eating Patterns[5]

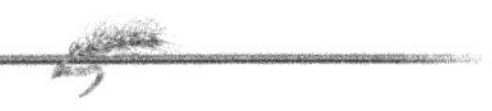

The plan below lists examples for a healthy U.S. food pattern at the 2,000 calorie level. The three examples show combined meals and snacks to meet daily food group intake needs: Fruits 2 cups; Vegetables 2½ cups; Grains 6 ounces (at least 3 ounces whole grains); Protein Foods 5 ½ ounces; and Dairy 3 cups.

Breakfast
1 ounce Grains
½ cup Fruit
½ cup Dairy

Breakfast
1 ounce Grains
1 cup Dairy
1 ½ ounces Protein Foods

Breakfast
1 cup Fruit
1 cup Dairy

Morning Snack
1 ounce Grains
1 cup Fruit

Morning Snack
1 cup Fruit
½ cup Dairy

Morning Snack
1 ounce Grains
½ cup Dairy
1 ½ ounces Protein Foods

Lunch
2 ounces Grains
1 cup Vegetables
½ cup Fruit
1 cup Dairy
2 ½ ounces Protein Foods

Lunch
2 ounces Grains
1 cup Vegetables
½ cup Dairy
2 ounces Protein Foods

Lunch
2 ounces Grains
1 cup Vegetables
1 cup Dairy

[5]https://www.cnpp.usda.gov/sites/default/files/usda_food_patterns/SampleMealPatternsForTheHealthyUS-StyleFoodPatternAtThe2000KcalLevel.pdf

Afternoon Snack
½ cup Vegetables
½ cup Dairy

Afternoon Snack
1 ounce Grains
½ cup Vegetables

Afternoon Snack
1 ounce Grains
½ cup Vegetables
½ cup Dairy
2 ounces Protein Foods

Dinner
2 ounces Grains
1 cup Vegetables
1 cup Dairy
3 ounces Protein Foods

Dinner
2 ounces Grains
1 cup Vegetables
1 cup Fruit
1 cup Dairy
2 ounces Protein Foods

Dinner
2 ounces Grains
1 cup Vegetables
1 cup Fruit
2 ounces Protein Foods

Appendix 6
Food Exchange List[6]

Vegetables contain 25 calories and 5 grams of carbohydrate. (One serving size equals 1 cup raw vegetable or salad, ½ cup cooked vegetable, or ½ cup vegetable juice.)

Fruits contain 15 grams of carbohydrate and 60 calories. (One serving size equals 1 small apple/banana/orange/etc., ½ grapefruit, 1 cup fresh berries/melon cubes, 4 ounces unsweetened fruit juice, or 4 teaspoons jelly/jam.)

Very Lean Protein choices have 35 calories and 1 gram of fat per serving. (One serving size equals 1 ounce of meat.)

Lean Protein choices have 55 calories and 2–3 grams of fat per serving. (One serving size equals 1 ounce of meat.)

Medium-Fat Proteins have 75 calories and 5 grams of fat per serving. (One serving size equals 1 ounce beef/pork chop, whole egg, or 1 ounce Mozzarella or other white cheese.)

Fat-Free or **Skim Milk** contain 90 calories per serving. (One serving size equals 8-ounces of milk or equivalent milk source.)

Starches contain 15 grams of carbohydrate (plus 3 grams protein and 1 gram fat) and 80 calories per serving. (One serving size equals 1 slice bread, ½ hamburger bun, ½ cup pasta, 1/3 cup rice/couscous/legumes, ½ cup corn/sweet potato/green peas, or 3 ounce baked sweet/white potato.)

Fats contain 45 calories and 5 grams of fat per serving. (One serving size equals 1 teaspoon oil/butter/mayonnaise, 1 tablespoon salad dressing/cream cheese, 8 large black olives, 10 large stuffed green olives, or 1 slice bacon.)

[6]Source: NIH National Heart, Lung, and Blood Institute: Aim for a Healthy Weight. https://www.nhlbi.nih.gov/health/educational/lose_wt/eat/fd_exch.htm#5

Appendix 7

Effect of Obesity on Health[7]

People who have obesity, compared to those with a healthy weight, are more likely to develop serious diseases and health conditions. Many of the following conditions may be more prevalent in the overweight/obese and can be helped by losing weight.

- Shorter life span
- Increased risk for coronary heart disease (CHD) according to the American Heart Association
- Stroke. Obesity places a strain on the circulatory system which can result in stroke.
- High blood pressure. Three out of four diagnosis of hypertension relate to obesity. High blood pressure increases risks for CHD, congestive heart failure (CHF), stroke, and kidney disease.
- Increased LDL cholesterol, lower HDL cholesterol, and higher levels of triglycerides
- Type 2 diabetes. Nine out of ten people with newly diagnosed type 2 diabetes are overweight. Type 2 diabetes nearly doubles the risk of death.
- Gallbladder disease

[7]Adapted from: Center for Disease Control:
https://www.cdc.gov/healthyweight/effects/index.html
National Heart Lung and Blood Institute:
https://www.nhlbi.nih.gov/health-topics/overweight-and-obesity

- Respiratory problems. More than half of those with obesity have obstructive sleep apnea.
- Osteoarthritis
- Mental disorders such as depression, anxiety, and others
- Body aches and pains
- Certain cancers

Appendix 8
Guidelines to Control Emotional Eating

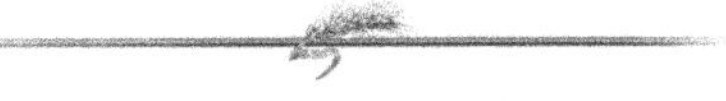

Observe yourself

- When you feel an urge to eat between meals, ask yourself if you are hungry and why you have a desire to eat.
- Become conscious of your eating behavior when you become angry, sad, or overcome with other emotions.
- Observe the time of day or situations that cause you to want to emotionally eat.

Develop coping skills

- Find reliable information about managing stress. Check for online articles, books, or other means.
- Share your feelings with a close friend who understands your situation.
- Take a walk or exercise to get your mind off food and rationally evaluate the cause of stress in your life.
- Occupy your mind with a hobby, book, or an interesting activity.

Value yourself

- Identify and make a list of your strengths and weaknesses.
- Focus on your value as a person.
- What interests you most and how often do you take part in that interest? Spend more time doing what you enjoy.
- What do you consider your greatest achievements in life (family, work, volunteerism, etc.)?

Appendix 9
Managing Chronic Stress

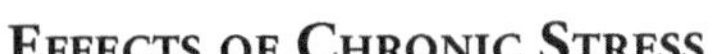

Effects of Chronic Stress

- Chronic stress seems to elevate ghrelin, an appetite-stimulating hormone found in the stomach.
- Ghrelin increases the desire for high-fat, high-sugar foods.
- The brain needs more and more hormone (ghrelin) and calming foods to obtain a mood change.
- Chronic stress causes more fat to be stored in the abdominal area, resulting in an apple-shaped figure. Those with more fat stored below the waist, pear-shaped, aren't as prone to as many disease conditions as their apple-shaped friends who are susceptible to increased risks for diabetes, heart disease, and cancer.

Tips for Tackling Chronic Stress

- Find a diversion—work a crossword puzzle; enjoy a hobby or favorite pasttime; walk outside for a few moments; walk away from the cause of stress for a short time.
- Head to the water fountain—drink more water, even if you aren't thirsty.
- Try to find one positive aspect in the situation—give thanks that the situation isn't any worse.
- Think—consider why you plan to use food for the stressful moment.
- Postpone indulging in food for 10 minutes. If still tempted, consciously decide to wait another 10 minutes.

Appendix 10
Binge Eating and Food Addiction

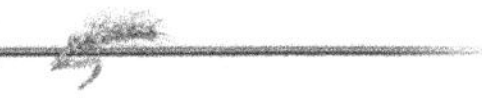

Binge Eating

Infrequent cravings do not necessarily result in a binge eater or a food addict.

A binge eater usually possesses the following characteristics:

- Eating much more in a short period than what is considered normal
- Out-of-control eating at least twice a week for a six-month period
- At least three of the following eating characteristics during binging episodes:
    - Eating more rapidly than usual
    - Eating until uncomfortably full
    - Eating large amounts of food when not hungry
    - Feeling embarrassed to eat with others because of the amount eaten
    - Becoming depressed, guilt-ridden, or disgusted with self

Food Addiction

Compulsive eaters who use food as a coping mechanism may develop compulsive/additive disorders resulting in negative behavior.

- Causes
    - Stress
    - Family history
    - Psychological problems (depression, low self-esteem, compulsive behavior)
    - History of abuse
    - Mood altered by the addicted substance
- Symptoms
    - Uncontrollable eating
    - Secretly binging
    - Feelings of guilt
    - Emotional eating
    - Social life affected by weight

Appendix 11
Choosing a Weight-Loss Diet

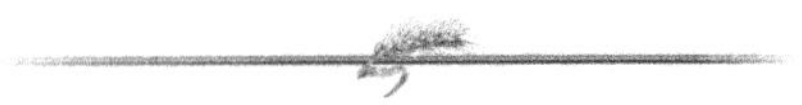

When it comes to weight loss, encouragement plays a vital role. One of the leading diets, WW (Weight Watchers), has succeeded in part because it encourages fellow members to meet and encourage one another. While there are many diets on the market, the U. S. News & World report for 2019[8] gave this diet high marks in several categories. It ranked number four out of a total of 40 diets in Best Diets Overall and tied for number five for Best Diets for Healthy Eating. When it comes to weight loss, this diet fared even better. The news magazine ranked it number one in Best Weight-Loss Diets and Best Commercial Diets. It tied for number two in Best Fast Weight-Loss Diets and Easiest Diets to Follow. These scores speak a lot about the quality of this diet.

While it is not the intent of this book to recommend specific diets, based on the scoring of experts in the fields of nutrition and health, this diet is worth investigating as you choose a safe and reliable diet to shed those extra pounds.

[8]https://www.usnews.com/info/blogs/press-room/articles/2019-01-02/us-news-reveals-best-diets-rankings-for-2019

Appendix 12
Tips for Cutting Calories

Change your snacks

- Instead of salty, sweet, or fatty choices, consider fresh fruit, air-popped corn, or nuts. While nuts do have more calories than some foods, in small quantities they provide many needed nutrients and a feeling of fullness.

- Cut one high-calorie treat daily. You choose. Is it the high-calorie breakfast doughnut, the tempting dessert at lunch, or fried foods?

Choose drinks with fewer calories

- Those special coffees or sugar-laden colas quickly add 400 to 500 calories a day—and leaves you without adequate nutrients or the needed fiber for lasting fullness.

Skip seconds

- When you can't resist, choose lower calorie foods. Instead of family style meals, serve buffet style without options for "all-you-can-eat" return trips to help the entire family control calories.

Substitute lower calorie ingredients in favorite recipes for high-calorie ones

- Using plain low-fat yogurt instead of sour cream can cut a few hundred calories. Sugar can be reduced in many dishes without any effect on the results.

Say "no" to fried foods

- Save as many as 500 calories when you choose baked, broiled, or grilled foods instead of fried. Change those French fries to a baked potato, salad, or vegetable.

Build a thinner pizza

- An occasional splurge may be okay, but keep it minimal. Change the topping instead of skipping altogether by omitting the cheese and meat and load your pizza with lots of veggies.

Eat from a plate

- Put smaller portions of favorite snacks, like regular popcorn, chips and other tempting snacks on a plate or in a bowl. When it's gone, it's gone. Avoid grabbing sandwiches and bags of chips on the way to the TV. Most tend to eat less when meals are placed on a plate and eaten in a designated area away from distractions.

Avoid alcohol

- While that isn't a problem for many, it is for some. Alcohol has no nutritive value but lots of calories. Some drinks have as many as 500 calories. For those who choose to drink, light beers or a small glass of wine have fewer calories.

Use smaller plates at meal time

- Perception of the amount of food is greater on a small plate than the same amount placed on a large plate.

Make it a point to eat your meals at the same place daily

- When at home, eat at the same place (table, eating bar) to establish a pattern of where to eat.

Don't skip breakfast

- The same number of calories eaten earlier in the day seems to have a better weight effect than when eaten later in the day.

Appendix 13
Tips for Eating Out

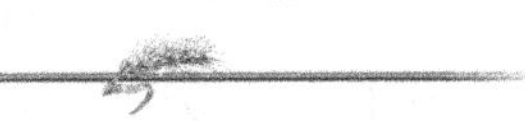

- Order red sauces instead of white to lower calorie intake.
- Request all dressings, sauces, butter, and gravies be served on the side so you can control serving size. Then use sparingly.
- Choose entrees of chicken, seafood, or lean meat instead of fatty meats.
- Check for menu items marked "healthy." Choose steamed, broiled, baked, grilled, poached, or roasted foods instead of those fried, smothered, sautéed, creamed, or au gratin.
- Avoid cocktails, appetizers, and bread and butter before the meal.
- Avoid all-you-can-eat buffets and specials. Order from the menu or discipline yourself not to return for seconds.
- If you choose high-calorie foods, i.e. pizza or sweetened beverages, order the smallest size.
- Split orders with someone else, ask for smaller portions, or ask for a to-go box at the beginning of the meal to help control the amount you eat.
- Resign from the "clean-plate-club." When you begin to feel full, stop eating.
- Change sugary beverages to no-calorie drinks and choose low-fat dairy products.

- If you usually order both sour cream and butter for a baked potato, make a choice, pick only one. Or make a conscious choice to use half the amount of each.

- Check the menu for calorie counts. National food chains are required to list the number of calories by items. Choose those lower in calories.

Appendix 14
Nutrients for Good Health

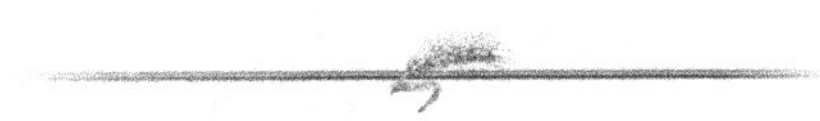

Energy Nutrients

Our bodies need energy (fuel) in the form of calories. Energy or calories for our bodies come only from carbohydrates, proteins, and fats. An ounce of fat provides more than twice as many calories as the same amount of carbohydrate or protein (which have about the same). The calories we need depend on age, activity, gender, and other factors. Healthy adult women of appropriate weight need about 2,000 calories a day. Men and very active women need more while older people need fewer.

Vitamins

These nutrients help change carbohydrates, fats, and proteins into energy, carry out body functions within the cells, and form bones, teeth, and tissue.

Minerals

Mineral elements help regulate enzymes, build body and bone tissue, and keep nerves and muscles healthy.

Water and Fiber

Both water and fiber help in losing weight and maintaining weight loss. Drink ample fluids (six to eight glasses each day), especially water. Foods high in fiber help eliminate waste from the body.

Phytochemicals

This chemical substance, found in plants, derived it name from the Greek work "phyto" which means plant. Unlike vitamins and minerals, these aren't essential to keep one alive, but they help prevent diseases and keep the body functioning properly. Major sources include fruits and vegetables along with whole grains, nuts, tea, and beans.

Appendix 15
Common Medications and Weight Gain

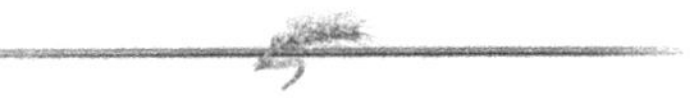

Modern medicine has kept us well longer and increased our lifespan. Most medications have some potential for side effects, and package inserts give that information in addition to dosage and other relevant facts. Drugs are prescribed to treat conditions to keep us healthier and functional. Reactions and dangers exist when certain medications are stopped abruptly, so none should ever be discontinued without discussing with the physician who prescribed it.

Weight gain

Increases in weight can result from several factors, especially as we age. Not all medications with weight gain listed as a side effect will cause all patients to gain weight since drugs may affect people differently. While most extra weight results from eating more calories than we use up, other situations can contribute. Some medications may cause fluid retention, decreased activity/tiredness, or increased appetite, all a possible cause for gaining weight. Common drugs that may lead to weight gain include:

- **Antidepressants.**
- **Antihistamines**. May result in increased appetite. Common over-the-counter (OTC) drugs include Zyrtec and Allegra.
- **Antipsychotics/Mood disorder.** Some drugs for mental health conditions may increase weight by as much as 7 – 10 percent.

- **Blood pressure.** Beta blockers may cause fatigue in some patients and result in less activity to burn calories. Calcium channel blockers and ACE inhibitors are less likely to cause weight gain.

- **Diabetes medications.** Some drugs can increase appetite. Others may result in fluid retention. Metformin, a common choice of medication, is not related to weight gain.

- **Pain/inflammation – corticosteroids.** Oral corticosteroids increase the risk of weight gain when taken in high doses or for long periods of time. Steroids, such as prednisone, can affect the metabolic rate and lead to increased appetite and overeating. Injectable corticosteroids are not linked to weight gain.

Appendix 16
Seven Principles for a Healthy Diet

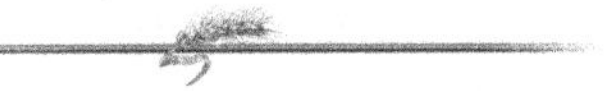

We all eat. We can't survive unless we do. Food is not the enemy—even high-calorie choices have their place. Likewise, diet is not a bad word. We all are on a "diet." The word refers to whatever we eat—from toast and water to caviar and wine—that is our diet. Small changes can drastically alter a less healthy meal pattern into one that helps maintain a healthy weight and improve overall health.

- Avoid high-fat, high-sugar foods and keep them out of the house to prompt more healthful eating and loss of weight. Sugar doesn't need to make us fat. It's that huge amount we tend to add to foods and drinks.
- Add instead of subtract. So-called "weight-loss diets" focus on what not to eat. Instead, consider what you can add to make your diet more healthy.
- Add fiber to ensure a greater sense of fullness.
- Drink ample water between meals to keep you hydrated and replace some of the urge to eat.
- Add appropriate foods currently missing from your daily diet; five to seven servings of fruits and vegetables, four to six ounces of protein foods (lean meats, seafood, eggs, nuts, legumes), the equivalent of three servings of reduced-fat milk/milk products, and six servings of bread/cereal/pasta with half of those servings from whole grain sources. Use some of the above foods to make reduced-calorie desserts such as puddings or fresh fruit combinations.

- Watch portion size. One of the greatest culprits in the "battle of the bulge" is overindulgence. The following serving sizes help prevent consuming too much: fruits and vegetables, one-half cup cooked or one cup fresh; lean meats, about the size of a deck of cards; bread, cereal, or pasta, one slice or one ounce; milk/milk products, the equivalent of eight fluid ounces.

- Eat more slowly to bring about satiety and curb overeating. It takes about 20 minutes from the time food reaches the stomach for the brain to realize you are getting full.

Appendix 17
Reliable Internet Links for Promoting Good Nutrition

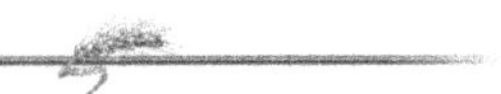

- Nutrition.gov: A USDA-sponsored website that offers credible information for making healthful eating choices **https://www.nutrition.gov/**

- Mayo Clinic: Reliable information on nutrition, healthy eating, physical activity, and food safety for consumers **https://www.mayoclinic.org/healthy-lifestyle/nutrition-and-healthy-eating/basics/nutrition-basics/hlv-20049477?reDate=31102016**

- Academy of Nutrition and Dietetics: A website for and by credentialed dietitians providing reliable information for professionals and consumers **www.eatright.org**

- American Heart Association: A reliable source for heart-related information, including diet **www.heart.org**

- American Diabetes Association: A website focused on those with diabetes that provides nutrition information as well as recipes **https://www.diabetesfoodhub.org/**

- National Institutes of Health-Aim for a Healthy Weight: Provides guidance and tools on how to make lifestyle changes to eat right **https://www.nhlbi.nih.gov/health/educational/lose_wt/eat/index.htm**

- American Cancer Society: Touts benefits of good nutrition, regular physical activity, and maintaining a healthy weight **https://www.cancer.org/healthy/eat-healthy-get-active.html**

- 2015-2020 Dietary Guidelines for Americans: Updated every five years, to help all Americans choose healthy eating patterns **https://health.gov/dietaryguidelines/2015/resources/2015-2020_Dietary_Guidelines.pdf**

- WebMD: Promotes itself as "The leading source for trustworthy and timely health and medical news and information. Providing credible health information, supportive community, and educational services by blending award-winning expertise in content, community services, expert commentary, and medical review." **https://www.webmd.com/**

www.ingramcontent.com/pod-product-compliance
Lightning Source LLC
Chambersburg PA
CBHW030246030426
42336CB00009B/277

* 9 7 8 1 7 3 3 7 0 5 2 0 2 *